*Medical Thinking:*
A *H*istorical *P*reface

# MEDICAL THINKING
## A Historical Preface

LESTER S. KING, M.D.

*Princeton University Press*
*Princeton, New Jersey*

*The medical texts of the 16th and 17th centuries,* and frequently of the 18th, were long and rambling. An impatient modern critic might say, "The older writers did not know much about science and so they filled their pages with harmless speculations; whereas today," the critic might continue, "we no longer have time for such leisurely word-chopping."

If, however, we actually read some of the older texts we find scattered discussions of quite fascinating topics: the nature of health and disease, the best way to classify diseases, the meaning of "signs," the nature of causation. Not, mind you, "the" cause of this or that disease, for such specific details have always been part of medical lore, but the nature of the causal relation in general. These topics—and there are many more—are conspicuously absent from our modern texts of medicine.

The modern critic might say that now these and similar topics are all part of the flourishing discipline we call philosophy of science, and with great satisfaction he can point to university departments that specialize in such matters. He might add that beginning in the 19th century physicians concentrated on the substantive topics in science, while subjects with a philosophic tinge aroused little interest in the medical profession. To this generalization there have been noteworthy exceptions, such as Claude Bernard (1813-1878) or Sir Clifford Allbutt (1836-1925). Yet for the most part the broadly abstract concepts of medicine had been handed over to philosophers of science.

In the past fifteen years, however, the interest in medical abstractions has greatly increased and many relevant studies have emerged from quite diverse disciplines, to focus on the foundations of medicine. The interests of the more scholarly 17th-century physicians might seem to be slowly coming to life again. In the present book I try to hasten this process of revivification, and in so doing to show the essential unity of medical thinking throughout the centuries. I try to present a coherent if limited account of certain basic and recurrent ideas in medicine. Since my views derive from my entire medical background, a brief autobiographical note may clarify my particular approach.

In college I majored in philosophy. In medical school I developed a special interest in research on the nervous system. After an internship I engaged for almost seven years in pure medical research, in anatomy and pathology. Then, for almost twenty-five years I combined research with the practice of pathology. (The pathologist practices medicine and faces all the agonies of diagnostic decisions, even though he does not have the responsibility for treatment.) Then for the subsequent sixteen years, until my retirement, I was a medical editor and my contact with medicine was more indirect than it had been earlier. In medical history I have always been an amateur, in the sense that I have never depended on this discipline for my livelihood. However, for well over twenty-five years I have devoted a great deal of time to the subject, with adequate recognition from the professionals in the field.

In examining present-day problems I have tried to integrate my entire background: a concrete knowledge of medicine in both its investigative and diagnostic aspects, a philosophic training, and a command of medical history. My conclusions derive from the perspective thus gained.

This book is, in a sense, an *apologia pro vita mea*, while at the same time it is a preface to medicine—my views on what medicine is all about. It is the book I wish had been available to me some fifty-five years ago, when I first thought of studying medicine as a career. I am fully aware that the presentation is fragmentary, for I deal with only a few ideas and these in only partial fashion. Any one of the chapters could easily be expanded into an entire monograph—if several lifetimes were available.

In my retirement I appreciate more than ever the lines of Robert Browning:

Ah, but a man's reach should exceed his grasp.

And conscious of the imperfections in this book I would again quote Browning:

What I aspired to be,
And was not, comforts me.

It is with great pleasure that I give special thanks to Miss
Cecile E. Kramer, librarian at the Northwestern University
Medical School, for the privilege of using that splendid library.
I thank also the library staff of the American Medical Association, who have been unfailingly helpful. And I must make
grateful acknowledgment of the financial aid from Grant LM
03157, of the Department of Health, Education, and Welfare.

# TABLE OF CONTENTS

PREFACE                                                                    V

## BY WAY OF BACKGROUND
Chapter 1   *Persistent Problems of Medicine*                               5
Chapter 2   *Consumption: The Story of a Disease*                          16

## SOME BASIC CONCEPTS
Chapter 3   *Signs and Symptoms*                                           73
Chapter 4   *Diagnosis*                                                    90
Chapter 5   *Classification*                                              105

## DISEASE
Chapter 6   *Disease and Health*                                          131
Chapter 7   *The Clinical Entity and the Disease Entity*                  146
Chapter 8   *When, Where, and What Is the Disease?*                       165

## CAUSE
Chapter 9   *The Causes of Disease: I*                                    187
Chapter 10  *The Causes of Disease: II*                                   204

## TREATMENT
Chapter 11  *Reflections on Blood-Letting*                                227

## HOW DO YOU KNOW?
Chapter 12  *What Is a Fact?*                                             247
Chapter 13  *The Scientific Method, So-called*                            267
Chapter 14  *"Scientific Medicine"*                                       294

EPILOGUE                                                                  311
NOTES                                                                     319
INDEX                                                                     331

*Medical Thinking:*
*A Historical Preface*

*BY WAY OF BACKGROUND*

———————◁ ▷———————

## CHAPTER I

# Persistent Problems of Medicine

## I

*In 1928, when I entered medical school,* our class was fully aware of the great ferment taking place in medicine. Insulin had only recently been discovered, and so had the curative value of liver in pernicious anemia. Endocrinology was emerging as an active discipline. The important role that electrolytes played in health and disease was receiving abundant study. Protein chemistry was making great progress, as was immunology. Surgical interventions were becoming more and more dramatic. By the time we graduated we were fully convinced that the medicine of our day was a truly scientific discipline and that it contrasted markedly with the empirical approach that had prevailed in the previous generation.

In the medical records that we wrote as students we would note the diagnoses and treatment that the patient might have received earlier from his family physician. We referred to this family doctor as the LMD—the local physician of the community, in contrast to the hospital-based physician—and we implied, condescendingly, that before the patient came into our hands he had been subjected not to scientific study but only to blundering guesswork. In the exuberance of youth we had little appreciation of the real problems of medicine.

The years passed swiftly. During World War II we were the young well-trained physicians, ten years out of school, rapidly becoming leaders in the profession. The book learning we had acquired seemed to remain essentially valid, and our theories had been tempered by considerable practical experience. During the war, and for a brief period thereafter, we enjoyed a sense of mastery that we would never feel again.

Our own training had taken place during economic depression, when research was receiving only limited support, and during war years, when research was more practical than theoretical. Then, after the war, medicine acquired a new momentum that increased at a frightening rate. For a long time the physicians of my generation could keep up in our own specialties and even contribute to their advancement. But as the years passed the over-all changes in both theory and practice forced each of us deeper into his own niche of specialization. And from our limited positions we could see a tidal wave of progress—new technology, new theory, new practice—engulfing the medical world. Younger men were taking over leadership. The years passed more and more rapidly until at length the members of my own generation could, if lucky, assume the status of elder statesmen in medicine. If not so lucky they acquired the status of old fuddy-duddy, regarded by the new bright young men just as we had regarded the LMD who had graduated in 1905 or 1910.

The great rush of progress produced the viewpoint that modern medicine differed markedly from that of the past, and that only now, in what we may call the electronic age, was medicine at last *really* scientific. And the questions arose: When did this transformation take place? When did medicine become truly modern, truly scientific? In 1932 my own generation thought that it had all the answers, but now the new generations of physicians, together with the students they taught and the lay public they indoctrinated, all had a different set of answers. The very brash would say that only for the past ten years was medicine truly scientific, the more conservative would say twenty or twenty-five years. But there was general agreement that what took place more than twenty-five years ago was no longer part of current medicine but belonged rather to medical history. And what took place before World War II held only archeological interest for the medical student or resident. The general public tended to follow this belief.

This attitude was being continually reinforced by well-meaning deans and medical educators who would emphasize the transitory nature of medical education. In effect, these prophets said, of all the information learned today, approximately half would be obsolete within five years. Hence the catchy phrase, that the "half-life" of medical knowledge is a scant five years. Some optimists (or were they pessimists?) might extend the limit to as much as eight years.

Such concepts gave a vivid sense of tumultuous progress and appealed to the popular imagination. But for medical students this was a rather discouraging thought and for many of the older physicians twenty-five years out of school it was a shattering prospect indeed. But what does such facile generalization about medicine really mean? How much change have we actually had? Before we accept at face value all the publicity that medicine receives, we should study the presuppositions that inhere in the concept of medical progress.

The lay public shows a great curiosity about medical progress. Many newspapers and popular journals have special editors who ferret out the new discoveries and present the gist in suitable lay language. A constant stream of books and articles tells the public about the latest advances in medicine. To such lengths has popularization gone that physicians in practice occasionally complain that their patients, after reading popular magazines, may know more about new remedies than they themselves do.

This lay interest in health matters can distort our perspective. A succession of "breakthroughs," enthusiastically reported in the press, can lead the public to expect continued breakthroughs; and journalists looking for copy and not wanting to disappoint their public may magnify the importance of new medical reports. As a result, progress may seem to be greater than it actually is. Publicity may inflate significance.

Other factors may contribute to this inflation. Fund raising for medical research is big business, and fund raising thrives better when new advances seem imminent—hence the temptation to exaggerate the significance of new findings. Then, as a correlative, institutions that seek research support may sometimes encourage publication before conclusions are fully estab-

lished. And, among individual researchers, the race for priority
may induce premature publication or exaggerated claims. Without laboring the point I suggest that important advances may
not be as numerous as we may at first think.

Yet, even after allowing for exaggeration and inflated importance, we must stand in awe at the changes that have taken place
in medicine in the past twenty-five years. They affect all modalities. We have new modes of treatment, ranging from a
succession of "wonder drugs" to fabulous operations such as
microsurgery and organ transplants, while new diagnostic tools
such as computerized x-ray studies allow extraordinary discriminations. More important, however, are the conceptual advances
in fields as widely diverse as immunochemistry, neurophysiol-
ogy, and genetics.

Yet those who concentrate on advances in medicine lose sight
of an important truth: the very fact of change implies something
constant that does not change. Aristotle expounded this principle
when he distinguished form and matter. Forms do indeed
change, but the constant feature that does not change he called
"matter." In medicine today the Aristotelian doctrine of form
and matter does not have the significance it had 350 years ago,[1]
but the principle involved does have relevance. In the explosion
of medical knowledge we readily appreciate the facts of change—
they are vast and indisputable—but we must not ignore the aspects of constancy, those features of medicine which have not
changed. In our present-day preoccupation with what is new,
we can profitably keep in mind the factors that remain the same.


## II

Let us approach this problem indirectly, by considering the student who is just beginning the study of medicine. I suggest that
such a person is taking part, even if unwittingly, in a sort of
relay race. We can imagine an invisible runner, a shadowy representative of times gone by, who approaches the new student
and presses into his hand a scarcely palpable baton and then
vanishes back into the world of shades. The student at first is
perhaps not even aware of the baton he is carrying, but as he

gains experience and maturity this heritage from the past begins to take on a perceptible shape. In time, as the student acquires further insight, he will realize that the baton had undergone many changes from the many hands that had grasped it in the past. And before he himself can pass it on, his own hands will have moulded it into something different.

The metaphor of a baton will symbolize the heritage of medicine that passes from one generation to another. For easier discussion I suggest a threefold division of the total tradition. First is the heritage of knowledge, that is, the aggregate of information painfully accumulated, together with the theories derived therefrom. This knowledge gets embodied in textbooks. Since medical information and medical ideas undergo constant modification, doctrines are always in a state of flux. The many changes get recorded in texts and journals, whose contents show marked transformation from one generation to the next. A survey of successive doctrines would comprise a history of medical concepts through the ages. This part of our heritage has received a great deal of attention from historians, but for the moment we will pass it by.

The baton also includes a heritage of traditions, customs, and behavior. Here I include that broad area often called medical ethics, which indicates what conduct is right and what conduct is wrong, as physicians treat their patients and interact with their fellow physicians and with society. In a wider sense this aspect relates not only to professional behavior but to the entire social relationships of the physician, considered as a healer, as a citizen, and as a member of society. This tradition of medical behavior is in part parochial, in part bound to total morality.

The third division, and the one that concerns us the most, I would call the heritage of problems. Over the past twenty-five hundred years of medicine certain problems have persisted with remarkable constancy. The medical student can draw comfort from realizing that when he enters practice he will be facing essentially the same problems that his medical ancestors also faced. As they labored to find solutions, so he too will labor. We must distinguish, however, between the continuity of the problems and the variations in the answers. The answers change; the problems, the questions, remain the same.

What, then, are these questions which remain constant? There is no single canonical list, for any selection will depend to some extent on interest. However, in line with my own interests I offer several suggestions, each of which has its own ramifications and subordinate topics. What is the disease from which the patient suffers? How can we identify it? What can we do for it? How can we prevent it? What is its cause? How much confidence can we place in our assertions and our judgments? How do we know if we are right in what we say and what we do?

These questions sound deceptively simple, so much so that they may seem scarcely worth bothering about. Quite obviously they engage the attention of physicians today. And even the most anti-historical scientist will grudgingly admit that in times past physicians probably had similar concerns. But, he will say, the conditions are so different that no comparison is possible. He will stress not the problems but the answers and will want to attend to the changes that have taken place in medicine in the past thirty or one hundred or one hundred and fifty years. Indeed, so prevalent is this attitude that, when regarding the past, most physicians and most laymen concern themselves with the overthrow of past error, the exposure of absurdities, the succession of triumphant breakthroughs, the achievements of technology.

An enormous literature recounts the triumphs of modern medicine, and in so doing stresses the aspects of medicine that have changed over the years. Such an emphasis, however, completely distorts the nature of medical science and medical practice. This distortion manifests itself by creating sharp discontinuities and sudden breaks with the past. An example of this type of thinking we find in Lewis Thomas. His views, which I offer in some detail, represent the diametrical opposite of my own concepts of medical history.

In a chapter called "Medical Lessons from History,"[2] Thomas described the period of the 1930s when the sulfonamides and penicillin were discovered. This, although a "major occurrence" in medicine, he did not consider to be an actual revolution. "For the real revolution in medicine . . . had already occurred one hundred years before penicillin. . . . Like a good many revolutions, this one began with the destruction of dogma. *It was discovered, sometime in the 1830s, that the greater part of medicine was nonsense*" [italics added].

Pointing to the unpopularity of medical history, Thomas said, "And one reason for this is that it is so unrelievedly deplorable a story." For millennia, he claimed, "Medicine got along by sheer guesswork and the crudest sort of empiricism. It is hard to conceive of a less scientific enterprise among human endeavors." Earlier treatments he condemned as "the most frivolous and irresponsible kind of human experimentation, based on nothing but trial and error." He believed that the traditional remedies rested "on the weirdest imaginings about the cause of disease, concocted out of nothing but thin air—this was the heritage of medicine up until a little over a century ago. It is astounding that the profession survived so long and got away with so much with so little outcry. . . . Evidently one had to be a born skeptic, like Montaigne, to see through the old nonsense." There was, apparently, no merit in medicine until the 1830s. Then, for reasons that Thomas does not disclose, there occurred a sudden discontinuity and the real beginning of modern medicine.

These paragraphs indicate Thomas' attitude toward the medical past and toward medical history as a discipline. I quote him to show the views toward history of a prominent and influential member of the medical profession, with a wide popular following.

Interestingly enough, Thomas uses the same word "heritage" to which I attach so much importance. In his words the earlier heritage was "concocted out of nothing but thin air"; but apparently "a little over a century ago" the heritage started to take on substance and significance and led to modern medicine. This, in my view, is an absolute misreading of history, one that, among its other errors, pays attention only to the changes and ignores the continuities. In my view our medical heritage, for at least twenty-five hundred years, has shown a continuity, with a sub-strate that exhibits a remarkable constancy—namely, a constancy of problems. In this book, I will deal with some of the problems of the past as they continue to concern present-day medicine. The key to understanding the present lies with the past, and the study of the medical past comprises medical history.

## III

If I were to ask, "Of what use is a sledge hammer?" the answer would be quite easy. I could give a concrete example: a sledge hammer can, simply and directly, break up a rock or get rid of an obstruction. In the appropriate context nothing else can do the job quite as well. But if we ask the question, "Of what use is medical history?" we can no longer offer a simple direct an-swer. We would be dealing not with a tangible object that ef-fectively transmits physical force but with knowledge, some-thing abstract and intangible. No one would claim that a sound knowledge of Galen, for example, would make it easier for a surgeon to remove a gall bladder, comparable to the way that the use of a sledge hammer would enable a workman to break down a brick wall more efficiently.

If we replace the word "use" with the word "value," and rephrase the question to read, "What is the value of medical history?" we have somewhat more leeway. There is no longer any question of a "practical" effect and we are entering a quite different realm. The realm, however, is full of pitfalls, for it has to do with preference and choice, with judgments of good and bad, of better and worse.

Such judgments can arouse heated controversy. Are there any properties that make one activity *better* than the other? Can we find some context in which we can say, "In this particular situ-ation, a knowledge of medical history provides some special value and permits us to achieve a result *better* than we would have had without that knowledge?" Unfortunately the term "medical history" is itself hard to pin down. While there is nothing elusive about the characteristics of a sledge hammer, the history of medicine will mean different things to different people at different times. We can pass value judgments on medical history only when we indicate the sense that we attach to the term.

As recently as sixty years ago medical history was dominated by what I call old-line historians, great scholars, most of them German, who delved into the past and produced series of books that were for the average physician profoundly uninteresting. The medical historians, although they would talk fluently to each other, had little to say to a more general audience.

I speak feelingly on the subject, for when I was a first-year medical student I was subjected to lectures drawn from such scholarly texts. The lectures, punctuated with lantern slides, offered information of not the slightest interest to the students. The class reached a consensus: that one old gentleman with a beard looked very much like any other old gentleman with a beard. The lectures did not convey any sense of relevance to the subjects we were studying. To be sure, while we were dissecting a cadaver we found interest and even amusement in seeing pictures of Vesalius' "muscle men" in their odd postures. Yet, with such rare exceptions, the medical history to which I was exposed proved singularly unappealing.

There was no trace of "relevance." This word has since become a rallying cry of disaffected youth who want an excuse for not doing what they do not want to do, and who resent the attitude of educators that the older generation obviously knows best. Despite my natural ties with the (very much) older generation, I must sympathize here with the students. I defend the legitimacy of the questions, "Why is this important? What is the relevance?" When the questions are raised, the teacher should be able to answer them. He should at all times be ready to indicate the importance of what he teaches.

Importance I regard as a function of interest. The good teacher who arouses interest in his subject thus provides the framework whereon the data will take on relevance. Interest gathers strength when there is some congruence between the experience of the student and the events of the past. If we stress the differences between the past and the present, we destroy the sympathy that the student might have been able to build up. If, however, we can indicate the similarities between the past and the present—the similarities that persist through the obvious differences—we can induce a more sympathetic understanding.

These two different approaches we can exemplify by a reference to blood-letting. It is very easy for a lecturer to get an audience into good humor by recounting a few details about the horrors of blood-letting and the enormous excesses to which the patients were often subjected. The audience usually gets a message, conveyed with varying degrees of subtlety: "How lucky to live now, with the wonders of modern medicine, rather than in those old benighted days!" Medical history thus serves to enhance the modern ego and in so doing inhibits any sympathetic understanding with the past. The information is entertaining and ego-boosting, but there is no sense of relevance and the audience perceives no connection between the events of the past and those of the present.

On the other hand, the lecturer may explain what the older physicians were really trying to do, the problems they were facing, the concepts that guided their choices, and the tools they had to work with. He may indicate the parallelism to the present: just as today, the physician must treat the patient according to the available concepts and must use the available tools. The lecturer will, if he is thorough, point out the therapeutic excesses that occur in modern medicine that may be just as devastating as the analogous excesses of two centuries past. The lecturer who pursues such a course may convince the audience that the past is truly relevant to the present, despite the multiple differences.

If the physician remains limited by his own experience and by that of his immediate contemporaries, he has shut himself off from the accumulated wisdom of the past. This wisdom does not in any way deal with exotic remedies and superstitious procedures. It does not call for a return to the purges and blood-lettings of Benjamin Rush, or to the use of mustard plasters for pneumonia. The wisdom will consist in an enhanced *critical attitude* toward all aspects of medicine.

History can give the physician a new awareness of the dynamic forces at work in medicine, the interactions of social and economic pressures, of ambition and pride and complacency, of cultural and technological limitations. And he will realize that he is dealing not with antiquarian details but with living problems that his predecessors faced, such as he himself is facing. By appreciating the difficulties of the past, he can gain increased acumen in identifying the difficulties of the present. If, however, he ignores the past, or regards its mistakes only as a way to achieve greater self-enhancement, then he is, in effect, blunting the critical sense he might otherwise develop. A sharp mind is even more important than a sharp scalpel.

I do not want at this point to enlarge on the concept of critical acumen, for this will emerge gradually in the course of this book. As a first step in my presentation I will offer a single case history, a history of the disease tuberculosis. This provides a study in progressive discrimination, whereby first insights gradually became more penetrating through the accession of new knowledge and the influence of new factors. The history of tuberculosis shows well the gropings of earlier physicians who knew nothing about bacteria or immunology or biochemistry or microscopy and yet had to face urgent problems of diagnosis and treatment. We can study the thought processes of highly intelligent physicians who did not have either the concepts or the technical aids that we recognize as important for the problems they faced. We will study the way they coped with the difficulties and the ways in which these expanded. In my exposition I will emphasize the logic of the earlier explanations and therapies that, of course, must be judged only in their own context. The story of tuberculosis will also provide concrete details for many of the concepts that I discuss later in the book.

The leaders in medicine in times past were just as intelligent as the leaders today. If the old procedures and assertions seem absurd, we must not conclude that they *were* absurd. We may conclude only that we do not fully understand the context in which the older physicians worked. The historian should reconstruct the context so that the actions of the leading practitioners appear reasonable and bear a logical relation to the problems involved.

## CHAPTER 2

# Consumption: The Story of a Disease

*Recently, when I lectured to medical students* on the history of tuberculosis, I asked the class how many were familiar with the disease called consumption. Only about a third of the students raised their hands—an interesting commentary on medical progress. Once a medical term of high repute, "consumption" gradually became outmoded and in the middle of the 19th century it gave way to the more precise concept, "tuberculosis." The older nomenclature faded even from popular usage; it now sounds rather archaic, eliciting mostly a blank stare. In an earlier period, however, consumption was deemed a quite specific term with a clear meaning, and if we analyze this meaning and trace the changes it underwent, we gain considerable insight into the process of medical thought.

Until about thirty or forty years ago, the word "consumption" had at least some vogue and was synonymous with tuberculosis. But in the 17th and 18th centuries it still retained its literal meaning—an eating up of something. Consumption was an eating up of the flesh, a wasting away. Such "melting" of the flesh by itself was not specific; it merely formed part of wider patterns. Of the many patterns in which wasting occurred, one was the disease we now call tuberculosis.

Today, thanks to the exquisitely precise tools at our command, it is quite easy to identify this disease. Radiology, microbiology, and serology greatly simplify the work of the practicing physician, give him ready means for having first a high index of suspicion, and then for reaching virtual certainty in his diagnosis. Today, distinguishing tuberculosis from other diseases with which it might be confused—i.e., the process of differential diagnosis—is for the most part relatively easy. But the 17th-century physicians, although they faced the same need for reaching a diagnosis, could not rely on precise tools. They did the best they could with only their unaided senses to help them. In this chapter I want to study their modes of thought, the ways in which they sought assurances, justified their pronouncements, and explained their results. And we will note the course by which comforting assurance eventually came to pass.

I am not in any sense writing a history of tuberculosis, but I use this disease to illustrate the progression of medicine during the past three hundred or more years, and to indicate some of the factors that led to the increasing precision of thought. In this exposition I will present only a few key figures who illustrate those features which I deem especially important. To better indicate the development of our knowledge, I will divide the exposition into stages which, however, are not in any sense rigorous or absolute. There are continuous overlaps, but even an approximate division makes the task of analysis much easier.

## CLINICAL OBSERVATION

In the first stage the physician had little to work with. He had no technical aids to help him to reach a diagnosis or to achieve a better understanding. He could only listen to the complaints of the patient, evaluate the reported data, and then examine the patient in a superficial and cursory fashion, essentially limited to the surface of the body. Infrequently the physician might perform or watch an autopsy. In addition, there was a large corpus of accumulated knowledge contained in texts and learned treatises. The physician had to reflect on all the information, weigh the evidence available to him, compare it all with the accumulated knowledge of the past, and reach a conclusion resting on his best judgment.

Of course, at all times physicians have weighed the evidence and then used their best judgment to reach a conclusion. The difference between the past and the present lies not with the need for judgment but with the amount of knowledge the physician had and the critical sense that he used. These aspects did change with time, as we shall see.

To exemplify the first stage, which I call clinical observation, I will discuss two prominent physicians, Richard Morton and William Cullen.

*Richard Morton*

Richard Morton (1635-1698) wrote the first great work devoted entirely to consumption. The disease itself had been recognized by the ancients and had received at least some degree of attention from every important medical writer. But Morton, in 1685, produced a landmark study that profoundly influenced all later physicians. His book, written in Latin, was translated as *Phthisiologia: or a Treatise of Consumptions*. *Phthisis*, of course, is the Greek word for consumption, and the Latin equivalent at that time was *tabes*. The terms, with their English rendition, consumption, were interchangeable. Morton's usage—representative of his era—is reflected in the extended title: ". . . wherein the difference, nature, causes, signs, and cure of all sorts of consumptions are explained." The plural usage is a crucial feature—there are many kinds of consumption.[1]

Wasting of the body may be generalized, affecting the body as a whole, or localized. The latter category we can ignore. If we consider only patients with generalized emaciation, we note that some will show disease of the lungs, others will not. By definition both types represent consumption.

Many diseases produce generalized emaciation without involving the lungs in any destructive process. For example, we can have generalized wasting in severe diarrhea (the "bloody flux"), long-continued blood loss, diabetes, "dropsy," and chronic "weeping" ulcerations, among others. Obviously, not every patient with such ailments would go on to pulmonary consumption, but a sufficient number did to suggest that these wasting diseases might at times have some connection with pulmonary disease.

On the other hand, many patients became ill with true pulmonary consumption, without showing clear evidence of pre-existing disease. Morton, therefore, divided the cases of pulmonary consumption into two major classes, the primary, with no signs of pre-existing disease; and the secondary, which did show such signs. Morton's own terms, for this division, were "original" and "symptomatic," depending on the absence or presence of some other disease as precursor. Since his text offers a bad cross-classification that, if followed literally, leads to wordy confusion, I will pursue his key ideas rather than try to follow his exposition sequentially.

As Morton abundantly showed, wasting of the body could occur regardless of whether or not the lungs were involved in any disease process. To account for the wasting, as such, he blamed faulty nutrition. There might be a lack of nutritious chyle (i.e., the soupy product of digestion that gets absorbed from the intestine); or the chyle was unfit for nourishment; or the lack of proper chyle weakened or oppressed the spirits; or the blood could not assimilate the new chyle. He was saying, in different ways, that the wasting occurred because the blood could not, for whatever reason, bring nutritive material to the body.

Consumption of the lungs, in its fully developed state, was a distinct clinical entity. Morton offered three identifying features: a wasting of the whole body (in contrast to a merely localized atrophy), a hectic fever, and an "exulceration" of the lungs. This referred to the cough that at first was dry and non-productive but later would become purulent—i.e., productive—and resulted in cavities in the lung. When all these features were present, we had a case of pulmonary consumption—by definition. These features, present in every case of the disease, were sufficient in themselves to allow a diagnosis. And the physician could observe them at the bedside.

As we have seen, this form of consumption might appear as a primary disease or, if it followed some other ailment, would have a secondary status. Morton's chief interest lay in analyzing the way that the disease developed. What was its basic nature? What steps led up to it? Why did it attack one person rather than another? What were the causal factors? There were also the urgent practical problems: What is the best treatment? How can you prevent the disease? Let us study some of Morton's answers.

Morton recognized the great clinical variation in pulmonary consumption. Some cases, he showed, run a very acute course, proving fatal in a few months. Other patients have a long chronic course, live to an old age, and die of some unrelated ailment, even though they constantly show signs of their pulmonary disease. Patients get worse or improve—have exacerbations or remissions, to use the technical terms—under various circumstances. Can we specify these circumstances? Can we relate them to the symptoms, on the one hand, the bodily states, on the other? Any such explanation involves *theory*, and when a theory tells us how a disease comes about, we speak of pathogenesis.

Morton's theories of pathogenesis relied on traditional concepts of humors and qualities, and tried to integrate these with anatomical findings, on the one hand, with the symptoms, on the other. These aspects are strongly interrelated.

While Morton had at his command a store of traditional knowledge, his discussions were also informed by direct observation that could come only from a fair amount of autopsy experience. We have no idea of how many autopsies he performed or witnessed: the number in any case must have been minuscule when compared with the experience of the great French clinicians of the early 19th century. Nevertheless, although Morton did not advance the science of pathology, he did speak from firsthand knowledge and not merely from the reports of others.

In cases of phthisis the early physicians were quite familiar with the pathological findings known as the tubercle, a minute grayish lump often barely visible to the naked eye and usually ranging in size from a half millimeter to three or four millimeters. They may remain fairly localized or may spread, sometimes widely, sometimes to only a limited degree. Lesions originally discrete may become confluent, to form large masses. The central portions of the lesions ordinarily become necrotic, and when the lesions are large and the necrotic matter is coughed up, cavities will result. Morton was familiar with these gross findings. The cavities represented for him the "exulceration" that he regarded as a pathgnomonic sign of a "true" consumption of the lungs.

Today we know a great deal about this whole process. We know that the tubercle is the tissue reaction to the specific bacterium or to its products or constituents, and we know in great detail the tissue changes that may take place. We know the continuity between the early tubercles and the florid process of tissue destruction, with cavitation and death; or the slower course, with much fibrosis as healing tries to keep pace with destruction. We know the way in which the defenses of the body struggle against the infection and, if successful, bring about fibrosis, calcification, and clinical cure. We know a great deal about the phenomena that in the aggregate we call resistance and hypersensitivity, and we can explain them through detailed concepts of immunology and biochemistry. Morton, of course, had none of this knowledge, but he did have his own explanatory theories to account for the observations he was able to make.

As synonym of tubercle, Morton used the word "swelling," the English rendition of the Latin *tumor*. This swelling took place in the "glandules" of the lung, i.e., the alveoli or air-sacs. The tubercle arose, he thought, in the following way. A quantity of serum passed from the blood into the glandules of the lung and stagnated there, depending on the "thickness and glutinous quality of the lymphatick juice, that is separated in the glandules." The "parts"—the tissues—became distended, as a result of which they lost their natural "tone" and were unable "to spew or throw out the serum or water that flows into it." The humor—the exuded fluid—by degrees grew "dry and hard from the natural heat of the part" and this hardened serum constituted the tubercle.[2]

Morton knew that all exudations of fluid were not the same. He was fully aware, for example, that lobar pneumonia—the "peripneumonia" of the day—differed profoundly from a true consumption or the lungs. How to explain the difference? Wherein lies the specificity?

Unable to point to any material factors such as bacteria or antigens, he invoked different *qualities* of the blood or humors or temperament of the patients. In any given disease the blood could have a special quality from which the symptoms derived, whereas in some other disease a different quality obtained.

The special quality induced, somehow, the particular result. Among the qualities a favorite term was "sharpness." The humor that possessed a special sharpness would have different properties and potentialities from a humor that lacked that particular sharpness. So too with other qualities, such as hot or mild, or benign or malignant. These properties of a humor would determine the action in the body and affect the course of the disease.

A main factor was thus the "disposition of the blood, and of the humour which is supplied to the tubercles" and these dispositions will vary "according to the various dyscrasy [sic] of the blood." A malignant humor—one that is particularly sharp and hot—will produce a disease that runs a rapid course and is certainly mortal. If, however, the tubercles arose from "some benign, mild, and cold humour, such as is less apt for inflammation and putrefaction," then the patient will live longer. And if the mass is not at all "disposed to an inflammation and putrefaction, the distemper is very chronical" and the patient may live a very long time. This type of explanation, prevalent in the 17th century, formed part of the Galenic tradition that dominated medical thinking of the era. Elsewhere I have discussed these aspects at considerable length.[3]

Morton's terminology may seem at first glance merely to repeat in shorthand fashion the phenomena he is trying to explain. He did not show how one quality—invoked as an explanation—differed from another except in the result it produced. Yet before we condemn him we should think of our modern vocabulary and the way that modern medical theory invokes such terms as "virulence" and "resistance." If Morton had said that one humor was more virulent than another, he might have seemed closer to the modern idiom.

Consumption bore a special relationship to the tubercle. By itself the simple tubercle did no special harm. Its formation seemed to depend on non-specific factors: the passage of fluid into the lung spaces and later a drying out and hardening. As long as these little swellings remained in their original state— which, in Hippocratic terminology, Morton called crude—they might simply go away. Indeed, they usually did so, for, he said, they were so common, so widely found, that mankind would be destroyed if these little bodies did not readily disappear. The crude tubercle, then, as it derived from the blood, was entirely benign.

However, it was potentially dangerous. If an inflammation supervened, the tubercles could become malignant and destructive. This inflammation might have two causes, an internal and an external. The internal factor would be the sharpness present in the blood and exuded humor but quiescent. This sharpness, with its malignant property, might be incited into action by external factors. Morton illustrated this intermingling of factors: a frequent disposition to coughs, he said, suggests that a consumption of the lungs might be at hand. And this consumption "will most certainly seize the patient, whenever the serous part of the blood has contracted so great a sharpness as is sufficient to inflame or exulcerate the lungs, *either from the liberal drinking of spirituous liquors, or from taking of great colds or any other cause*.[4] Thus, the sharpness, the basic factor, could be made operative by various external factors that included disregard of hygienic living. Sharpness, when active, produces inflammation; the extrinsic or contributing factors—the disregard of hygiene—may be said to *induce* the inflammation and thus serve as activating factors.

This view ties in neatly with the recommended therapy. If the key factors are sharpness (with its related heat) and inflammation, then the proper treatment for threatened consumption would be to avoid excessive heat. Hence the physician must not use strong purges, for these throw the blood into excessive motion and can make it too hot. The physician should temper the heat of the blood through gentle laxatives that will "carry off the load of humors by stool gently, and by degrees." Similarly, in the early stage of the disease a moderate amount of bloodletting may "cool" the blood. An opiate will "quiet the lungs, which at this time are heated by the continual and violent motion of the cough," and also "calm the whole mass of blood." Heat and sharpness offered a reservoir of explanation.[5]

Before we leave Morton I want to mention briefly two conditions especially relevant to consumption: catarrh and scrofula.
Each of these was considered a disease in its own right, the one
an affection of the lungs, the other of the lymph nodes (or
"glands"). Their precise connection with phthisis troubled Morton and continued to trouble physicians until the last quarter of
the 19th century.

Catarrh represented what we call "bronchitis," manifested by
a cough that yielded abundant sputum. In its "simple" state it
was clearly separable from consumption, for the two diseases
affected different parts of the lung. Catarrh involved the trachea
and bronchi, consumption the "spongey" parts of the lung, i.e.,
the alveoli. A simple catarrh begins as a "distillation of rheum
cast out in continual drops by . . . glands seated in the upper
part of the wind-pipe, yea, and by all the glandulous coat of the
wind-pipe itself" (i.e., the mucous membrane). Catarrh thus
involved the mucous lining of the trachea and bronchi, and the
cough was produced by irritation from the secreted mucus
(rheum). This cough is "always at the beginning moist and
joined with a great flux of humours." In consumption, on the
other hand, the cough in the early stages is always dry (i.e.,
non-productive), for "it proceeds from a swelling of the lungs
rather than from any thin rheum owzing [oozing] out of the
internal membrane of the wind-pipe."[6]

In the early stages there is no difficulty in distinguishing simple catarrh from the cough of early pulmonary consumption,
but there may be great difficulty if the consumption is more
advanced and the cough no longer dry but productive. In theory
the differentiation between the two diseases was easy, but actual
practice was a different story. There was no reliable way to
decide whether the sputum contained only "rheum" or rheum
mixed with "corruption."

The second related disease that might induce confusion was
scrofula, the "King's Evil," for which the royal touch was
deemed curative. Today we know that this is a tuberculous infection that affects principally the lymph nodes, but in an earlier
period, when its nature was not clear, it was considered a sepa-

rate category of illness, identified on clinical grounds through "glandulous swellings in the external habit of the body . . . as also from an opthalmy [sic] or scab, that often returns. . . ." These characteristics seemed to distinguish it quite clearly from consumption of the lungs, with its cough, fever, and emacia- tion. Yet a child affected by scrofula would very often later develop true pulmonary consumption. And, conversely, some patients with florid phthisis might on autopsy show extensive swelling of the lymph glands, which were filled with a peculiar "chalky, or steatomatous substance."[7] Were scrofula and phthisis two phases of the same disease or two separate diseases, one of which might pass over into the other? Morton adopted the latter view.

Morton had superb clinical acumen and sound judgment. However, he had a limited amount of data with which to work, and he was laboring under an outmoded conceptual framework. The historian studies the way in which the data increase in amount, the conceptual framework slowly changes, and the pat- tern that we call a disease gradually takes on new boundaries. Morton serves as an excellent baseline for studying this process.

*William Cullen*

Morton we may regard as a pioneer who made a rough clearing in the forest. William Cullen (1710-1790), coming later, grubbed out many of the stumps and made an orderly planta- tion. The three-quarters of a century that separated Morton from Cullen brought about substantial changes in medicine. The physicians continued to observe their patients, theorize widely, and engage in lusty intellectual brawls. But in addition they sought regularity and order in their theories. Starting with a few basic concepts they tried to build comprehensive and sys- tematic doctrines to embrace all known medical data. The details of the various systems need not concern us here. However, this same passion for order also showed itself in the classification of diseases or, to use the technical term, "nosology."

In his discussions Cullen rarely used the term "consumption of the lungs" but preferred the synonym "phthisis pulmonaris" or more simply, "phthisis." He offered a precise definition: phthisis was an expectoration of pus or purulent matter from the lungs, attended with a hectic fever. This differs from Morton's definition in two major respects. Cullen's definition did not include emaciation, for in the early stages the diagnosis might be made before any wasting took place. Furthermore, since emaciation was a quite non-specific state, common to many diseases, placing it in the definition of phthisis could introduce ambiguity.

In further contrast with Morton, Cullen did not use ulceration of the lungs as a defining feature. Nosology depended on directly observable features. In the living patient the physician could not directly perceive ulceration of the lungs but could only infer it from what he did observe. Cullen made this distinction quite explicit. The cough was the symptom, but, since this was a feature common to many diseases, only a special kind of cough would indicate an ulcer of the lung, namely, a cough productive of "pus."

In the 18th century pus meant something quite different from what it means today. Now, thanks to our knowledge of microscopy and biochemistry, we define pus as a fluid or semi-fluid mass containing leukocytes, dead cells, and tissue debris liquefied through proteolytic enzymes of the white cells. Cullen, of course, had no inkling of these terms. He did know that pus meant tissue destruction that, if on the surface of the body, could be directly observed, but if inside the body could only be inferred. For him, then, the presence of pus served to indicate what might be going on out of sight.

However, pus that arose inside the body might not be easy to identify, not readily distinguishable from mucus. We have already seen that catarrh would have an expectoration of mucus. Said Cullen, "It has sometimes happened, that a catarrh was attended with an expectoration of a matter so much resembling pus, that physicians have been often uncertain whether it was mucus or pus, and, therefore, whether the disease was a catarrh or a phthisis."[8]

The one was a benign disease, usually self-limited, the other of the gravest import. A heavy responsibility thus rested on the physician who had to make the proper discrimination. Cullen indicated several ways to help him to reach a decision. The physician could observe the color and odor, and note whether the sputum sank in water—mucus usually floated; and he could test the reactions of the sputum to acids and alkalis, for pus and mucus behaved rather differently to these reagents. Here we have a true precursor of modern laboratory work and the use of "tests" to help a clinician reach a difficult decision. But these tests were by no means conclusive. They were suggestive only, and might help to tip the balance in a decision.

Of crucial importance was the fever. Many diseases had fever as a symptom; moreover, some diseases, such as catarrh or pneumonia, might also have cough and sputum. To derive any diagnostic value from the fever, the physician had to attend to its character. In phthisis this was of a special kind called "hectic"— occurring in the morning and again in the evening, with more or less remission in between. Another distinctive feature of hectic fever was the febrile flush that mantled the cheeks during the exacerbations, the so-called "malar flush." When the disease became more advanced, other signs would accompany the fever, but the hectic quality was a central feature in diagnosing phthisis.

The disease, thought Cullen, arose from an acrimony in the blood that, however, did not act directly on the tissues. Rather, it first produced tubercles, and these might then go on to ulceration, with the resulting symptoms. There were, he felt, different kinds of acrimony, any of which might produce tubercles. The acrimony in scrofula was probably similar to that in phthisis. Various exanthems like small pox or measles (often followed by phthisis) also had an acrimony that might produce tubercles—so too with syphilis, and probably other infections. Exposure to dust, Cullen noted, as among stone-cutters, could also lay a "foundation" for phthisis, "analogous, as I judge, to that of tubercles." He commented specifically on five distinct diseases that might give rise to hectic fever and to pulmonary phthisis. They deserve brief comment.[9]

First is hemoptysis, the coughing up of blood from the lungs. This may occur in various conditions, such as trauma or congestion, without any serious result, but sometimes the spitting of blood was followed by phthisis. Why in some cases and not in others? There must be some "particular circumstances" but what these might be "is difficult to determine." He invoked as a differential feature the body-build (e.g., a delicate physique and narrow chest), temperament, age, and many others. All these might help to distinguish those patients who would go on to contract phthisis from those who would not.[10]

Another disease often followed by phthisis was the abscess formation known as empyema that sometimes occurred in pneumonia. Ordinarily this complication of pneumonia would not lead to confusion, for, although there would be expectoration of pus, the fever was not hectic. Most cases of empyema did not go on to phthisis, but some did, and when this occurred, "it must be in consequence of particular circumstances which corrupt the purulent matter produced, render it unsuitable to the healing of the ulcer, and at the same time make it afford an acrimony." Any disease that seemed to result in phthisis acted by producing an acrimony that in turn produced tubercles.

Catarrh—the common cold or a simple bronchitis—was a quite benign disease, but on occasions it seemed to be a precursor of phthisis. When this happened, then in all likelihood "the persons affected were peculiarly disposed to phthisis." Or else there may have been a mistaken diagnosis, and what had been called catarrh was actually an early phthisis that had gone unrecognized.

Although asthma was commonly considered a cause of phthisis, Cullen dealt with this very briefly and believed that here too the mechanism took place by producing tubercles.

The most common causes of phthisis included hemoptysis, empyema, catarrh, and asthma, but most important of all was tubercle. Unlike hemoptysis, tubercle was not directly observed clinically but was noted only at autopsy. Then the physician might see "certain small tumors, which have the appearance of indurated glands." They may be indolent, but if they become

inflamed they get changed into little abscesses that "give a purulent expectoration, and thus lay the foundation of a phthisis."
Phthisis was one disease, and tubercle another disease that might
cause the former, or serve as its foundation.[11]

The term "tubercle" involved three shades of meaning: an
anatomical structure, observable at autopsy; a disease, comparable to catarrh; and a "foundation" for the disease phthisis.
This triple usage may confuse the modern reader.

A similar confusion attends the term "acrimony," which Cullen used to cover various situations. In different contexts the
same word might have varied reference—something that acted
on the tissues to produce tubercles; something responsible for
the clinical disease phthisis; something that derived from the
ulcers to prevent them from healing; or something that gave
rise to the particular hectic fever of phthisis. All of these meanings had a more or less genetic relation to each other, for they
all had to do with the same disease, phthisis. Other acrimonies,
of quite different character, related to other diseases and might
or might not have some connection with phthisis.

Cullen was trying to bring order into a confusing mass of
phenomena, and to do so he had to fall back on general explanatory concepts. He realized that he lacked precise knowledge,
for he was constantly hedging his comments with "probably" or
an equivalent. He relied on the vague concept of acrimony.
This, to our modern vision, was merely a catch-all. With the
further growth of knowledge during two hundred years, the
single vague concept became subdivided into several more precise terms, each of which served a portion of the total explanatory function.

## CLINICO-PATHOLOGICAL CORRELATION

In the history of tuberculosis I have called the first era the stage
of clinical observation (that is, study at the bedside) and I have
chosen Morton and Cullen as representative physicians. In the
three-quarters of a century that separated these men, the concepts of the disease became a little more refined, but no great
advance was made in understanding its nature. Progress was a

matter of degree rather than of direction. In modern jargon there was no breakthrough. Early in the 19th century, however, investigation underwent a distinct change in direction. At this point we may properly speak of a new stage, which I call the period of clinico-pathological correlation.

Over the centuries the post-mortem examination of patients with consumption had already provided much information. Indeed, only at autopsy could physicians have learned about the tubercle. In the early 19th century the number of autopsies performed increased greatly, but mere increase in number did not of itself mean much. The significance came from a new total approach, of which the actual autopsy was only a part.

To explicate, we must shift the scene to Paris in the first third of the 19th century. The Napoleonic era following the French Revolution had brought about social upheavals, cultural transformation, and rejection of traditional values and methods, and the momentum engendered thereby continued for many years after the fall of Napoleon. Young men with new ideas had been able to put them into practice without any chilling restraint of outworn conventions. This process of liberation had special scope in medicine. For our purposes I suggest as major factors the concentration of patients in the great Paris hospitals, and the opportunities for talented and hard-working young men to conduct painstaking studies along new lines. The physicians could observe large numbers of patients, become well acquainted with their clinical course, and then, if the patients died, correlate the clinical course with the autopsy findings. The important features were the large number of patients available for study, the care with which the disease was followed, the detailed post-mortem examination, and the tying together, for each individual case, of the anatomical and the clinical findings.

If we want, we can call this whole trend a new empiricism and contrast it with the rationalism of the 18th century. But empiricism and rationalism, although popular labels, are merely two aspects of a single process that seeks to achieve understanding. In the one case, special attention is paid to the data, in the other, to the inferences that result from the data. The difference is quantitative. How much data do we need in relation to how much inference? In the Paris school, so-called, the physicians accumulated quantities of data, both clinical and anatomical. But as a result of genius new inferences arose that I call a new insight—a breakthrough.

Many brilliant physicians worked in Paris during the first third of the 19th century—Bichat, Pinel, Bayle, Portal, Laennec, Louis, Broussais, to name only a few. Many of them contributed substantially to our knowledge of tuberculosis. However, I will attend mainly to Gaspard-Laurent Bayle (1774-1816), profound student of tuberculosis who himself succumbed to the disease at an early age, and to Laennec (1781-1826), also a victim of the disease.

## Gaspard-Laurent Bayle

To appreciate Bayle's contribution we must consider the question, "How do you know if the patient has phthisis?" Ordinarily we set up a definition (i.e., offer criteria), and then, if the patient conforms to that definition, we say that he has the disease. And, conversely, if the condition of the patient does not meet the criteria, we say he does not have the disease. Thus, to make a diagnosis we must have some sort of a definition, and definitions varied. For Morton, we have seen, the definition included emaciation. Cullen, however, knew that this was not essential, since consumption could be diagnosed before bodily wasting set in. Hence, he offered somewhat sharper criteria that involved only expectoration of pus and a hectic fever.

If the patient had an illness that did not meet the diagnostic criteria of phthisis, yet later developed that disease, then the first disease had been considered the precursor, or sometimes the cause, of the full-blown phthisis. In such a case there were supposedly two diseases, of which the first passed into the second. Especially important for the 17th- and 18th-century writers was the disease known as tubercle. We have seen that this was considered an important cause (or precursor) of phthisis.

Bayle brought about a marked shift in attitude. For him phthisis was not a disease that might appear rather suddenly, with or without precursors. Instead, it was a unified process that developed in stages over a time course, and the different stages might have quite different manifestations—i.e., symptoms. He offered a telling analogy, comparing phthisis to an oak tree. The mature oak would represent the florid disease. *But the seedling oak, while very different from the full-grown tree, is none the less an oak.* We must not refuse to call it an oak merely because it has a different appearance.

Similarly with phthisis. At its beginning the symptoms might seem trivial, scarcely more than a slight indisposition, yet it can progress to a massive ailment. *It is the same disease*, despite the variation in appearance. It has undergone a development. Physicians must learn to recognize the different stages, just as an entomologist must recognize different stages in the metamorphosis of an insect.

Hitherto the definition of the disease had been drawn from the florid stage, the result of pulmonary ulceration already well advanced. Bayle insisted that any definition should include the earlier stage as well as the later, and should reflect the progression. *Disease is process.*

To understand phthisis the physician must appreciate the process-as-a-whole, the "natural history" of disease. But this now had to include the pathological as well as the clinical aspects. Bayle's contribution, although extremely important, was brief and incomplete. In his book he distilled some of the insights he had gained from the autopsies he had performed. He identified six types of consumption, all of which showed a common pathologic factor. The patients need not have had fever or emaciation or purulent sputum. It was enough "if their lungs be affected by a lesion that leads to disorganization and ulceration." This is the first stage (*le premier temps*) of the disease phthisis, which, if it progresses, may lead to a fatal outcome.[12]

The *tendency* to disorganization was the key feature that distinguished consumption from other diseases of the lungs. The tendency—a dynamic concept related to process and development—could be identified by the anatomical changes in the lung. We learn the essence of phthisis by finding the organic basis for the symptoms, and by studying the way the progression of pathological changes paralleled the clinical appearance. The "essential character" of phthisis was more fundamental than the clinical manifestations. Morphologic changes underlay the signs and symptoms and were responsible for their appearance. This essence of the disease—its essential character—emerged through autopsy study.

Disorganization, although a vague term, is more or less synonymous with destruction. In his studies Bayle relied on gross observation alone, for at that time microscopy could offer no help. With only naked-eye observation, Bayle could identify certain types of lesions that would gradually progress to destroy the structure of the lung. Other diseases would behave differently. Catarrh, for example, an inflammation of the bronchi, was a benign disease that would not disorganize the structure of the lung. And neither would pneumonia, even though it might prove fatal. Tubercle, however, would disorganize the lung, although in some instances the patient might recover and die from some unrelated disease.

Bayle's six different types of phthisis produced the disorganization of the lungs in different ways. Most of the cases that he described—indeed, the overwhelming majority—were instances of tuberculosis, especially the types that today we call fibro-ulcerative and miliary. But in addition he included some other conditions that were non-tuberculous, such as those we now call anthracosis ("black-lung disease"), lung abscess, calcifications in the lung, and cancer.

We must realize, of course, that Bayle was describing not so much tuberculosis (which to us is a highly specific disease) but a more diffuse condition known as consumption (or phthisis). By seeking the *substrate that underlay the symptoms* Bayle tried to identify the essential character of the disease. But the disease that he was studying was not sufficiently clearcut. He had no notion of specific bacteria and no means of making microscopic differentiations. Relying only on gross observation he included several clinical conditions that fulfilled his criteria but that today, with different criteria, we recognize as different diseases. Bayle made a great step forward in discrimination. We must not complain that he did not carry his discriminations farther than his knowledge and techniques permitted.

As his great contribution Bayle directed attention to the pathology of phthisis rather than to the clinical features. Its essential nature lay in the pathologic changes. He laid special stress on the tubercle, whose gross appearances, distribution, and transformations he described carefully and well. Nevertheless, when he analyzed his various cases, he included several ailments that destroyed the lung tissues—and could therefore be called consumption—and yet had no intrinsic relation to the tubercle. He recognized the importance of the tubercle but not its essential role in any definition.

### René-Théophile-Hyacinthe Laennec

Bayle's work was amplified and corrected by his colleague and friend, René-Théophile-Hyacinthe Laennec (1781-1826). Laennec, widely known for his invention of the stethoscope, pioneered new methods of physical examination and probably did more than any other single physician to advance our knowledge of pulmonary diseases. His use of the stethoscope (and of percussion) enabled him to detect, through inference, what was going on inside the chest, hidden from direct sensory observation, and to correlate, while the patient was still alive, the clinical findings and the underlying pathology. Through his skill in physical diagnosis he could apply to the living patient some of the knowledge gained through anatomical studies.

Laennec's great book, *Traité de l'auscultation médiate* (1819), is one of the masterpieces of medical literature. It offered a profound analysis, both clinical and pathological, of diseases of the chest, including phthisis. This book appeared almost a decade after Bayle's work. Laennec fully acknowledged his debt to his colleague and friend, but in the intervening years he had learned a great deal more about phthisis. He extended the work of Bayle and in one major respect made a great advance.[13]

Laennec clearly realized the specificity of the tubercle and pointed out that Bayle's subdivision of phthisis into six species was untenable. There was the specific condition, "tuberculous phthisis," which might take more than one form. Other classes that Bayle had described, which we recognize as lung abscess, anthracosis, or cancer, had nothing essential in common with tuberculous phthisis. These other diseases did indeed involve the lung, and they might have a destructive effect—consumption in its literal sense. But in their essential nature they differed entirely from tuberculous phthisis and we should not include them under the same name.

Laennec used the unqualified term "phthisis" as the specific destructive disease of the lung uniquely associated with the tubercle, and the equivalent of what we now call "pulmonary tuberculosis." To Laennec we owe the rigorous correlation between the pathological structure known as the tubercle, and the clinical disease. Previously, phthisis was a term shared by several diseases. With Laennec it emerged as a clearcut entity whose natural history he did so much to clarify.

Other physicians of the Paris school further advanced our knowledge of the disease, but the contributions did not produce any additional breakthrough. This came only with the next stage, wherein gross observation was extended through the use of the microscope.

## The Contributions of Microscopy

As a clinical entity pulmonary consumption or phthisis was gradually becoming better defined. The French investigators had convincingly shown the close correlation between the disease and the tubercle, but the nature of the tubercle itself was not at all clear. The same name applied equally to nodules that differed in size, color, consistency, structure. They might be dry, crumbly, and granular, or moist and soft. The tubercle was often called pus. The tubercles, when large, might show central cavitation. At other times the tubercles might be firm and fibrous and even show calcific deposits.

Furthermore, in clinical phthisis structures resembling the tubercles of the lung might also be found in other organs, such as the lymph nodes, the surface of the brain, the intestines, the

peritoneum, and various abdominal organs. Moreover, these tubercles—or what seemed to be closely similar thereto—might
occur in diseases clinically quite distinct from phthisis, with
different symptoms and a different clinical course. Scrofula was
a prize example, whose relation to phthisis raised many persistent difficulties.

Did the variable appearances of the tubercle indicate different
diseases, or different stages of the same entity? As we have seen,
the earlier physicians believed the minute grayish tubercle posed
little hazard to health. But, so the contemporary theory went, if
the crude tubercle were overtaken by inflammation, it could
become malignant—spreading, ulcerating, and leading eventually to death. Here we have an additional problem: what was
the relation of tubercle to inflammation? The attempts to answer
these and kindred problems required an extension of knowledge,
and this came about through microscopy.

Today, with our excellent microscopes and refined histological
techniques, it is not easy to appreciate the difficulties that faced
the early workers. In the early compound microscope the resolving power was low, so that observers could not discriminate
between two closely apposed points or lines, which would be
seen as one, rather than as two. The lenses produced marked
spherical aberration, so that very small particles might appear
as globules, and fibers appeared as rows of globules. The images
as perceived did not reflect the real nature of the object under
examination. However, by 1827 spherical aberration was overcome. Continued improvement brought more and more precision, and by the 1880s the microscopes could provide excellent
resolving power, entirely comparable to the best light microscopes of today.

In the early days of microscopy there were no fixatives, no
microtomes for cutting thin sections, no staining methods for
revealing detail. Minute portions of fresh tissue might be
squeezed between pieces of glass, or fragments of tissue sliced
off free hand with a razor. Tissues were originally examined
fresh, unfixed, unstained, moistened by their own juices or by
a little water. A useful aid was dilute acetic acid, which seemed

to eliminate much of the debris and render some of the structures more clear than they had been. Solvents like ether might be added to dissolve some of the fatty material. Only well into the second half of the century were techniques developed for preparing thin sections with any degree of precision.

Before we take up the effects of microscopic study on our knowledge of pulmonary tuberculosis, I must note some of the terms that were prevalent, and clarify their meanings. I will discuss briefly the following concepts—cell, cellular tissue, blastema, vital activity, and organization. In the 19th century these terms had a meaning rather different from what they have today, and unless the differences are made clear the medical theories of the era will present an entirely false perspective.

## The Cell

In 1665 Robert Hooke published his *Micrographia*, one of the great landmarks of science. In it he described what he saw when he studied various common objects through his microscope. One of these objects was an extremely thin slice of cork. To his amazement it seemed "to be all perforated and porous, much like a honey-comb, but that the pores of it were not regular." He noted that "these pores, or cells, were not very deep, but consisted of a great many little boxes. . . ." These, he continued, "were indeed the first microscopical pores I ever saw," and, so far as we know, the first that anyone ever saw. And it also seems to be the first usage of the word "cell" in relation to biology.[14]

Unfortunately, many writers on medical history have confused the original meaning, of pore or cavity, with the modern usage that refers to the biological unit of life. As Baker points out, the modern concept of the cell evolved along two parallel lines, one concerned with plants and the other with animals. In the vegetable kingdom the cellulose walls, surrounding relatively empty space, in a fairly regular arrangement, made the term "cell" seem entirely appropriate. And indeed this designation for the microscopic appearance was so apt that it became well established even in the early literature.[15]

In animals the concept of the cell developed along rather different lines. The body fluids lent themselves much more readily to microscopic study than did the solids. Some time around the middle of the 17th century, observers, using the newly invented microscope, noted globules or corpuscles floating in the blood and other fluids. Minute fragments of solid tissues, when squashed and moistened, often showed comparable globules. Globules or corpuscles were found in a wide range of substances—in blood, milk, lymph, subcutaneous tissues, epidermis, glands, brain, feathers. The primitive instruments, coupled with the absence of staining techniques, did not permit sharp discrimination. There is often great difficulty for the modern student to know just what the older investigators were seeing. In many instances they were describing cells in our present sense, but in many instances they were referring to non-cellular material, such as fat droplets or tissue debris. The uncorrected lenses of the era prior to 1827 led to distortion and misinterpretation. Nevertheless, by the early 19th century a considerable amount of knowledge had accumulated, and the contemporary illustrations permit no doubt of the achievements.

Early observers also described the nucleus, in its modern sense, although they also used various other names, such as vesicle or clear body. Its presence would help to identify a cell and distinguish it from non-cellular material. By the 1830s the cell and the nucleus were terms quite current in the literature of anatomy and embryology.

How did the cells arise? What was their origin? Especially important for these questions is the work of Theodor Schwann (1810-1882), who published his major studies in 1838 and 1839. He was strongly influenced by his friend the botanist Schleiden, who was studying the growth of new-formed cells in plants. The process, thought Schleiden, took place *within* the relatively rigid walls of existing cells. Within the parent cell there was first formed a small structure that he called the cytoblast, corresponding to the nucleus. Upon the cytoblast grew the new cell, which appeared first as a delicate transparent vesicle, then got larger, and became individualized. Several cytoblasts could be formed free within a parent cell, which then was absorbed. The essential steps involved the formation of a nucleus within a parent cell and then the growth of new substance around the nucleus. Thus, a new individual makes its appearance.

Schwann studied animal tissue, beginning with notochord and cartilage, which, because of their firm texture, were relatively easy to manipulate and to prepare in thin slices. He believed that in these tissues the new cells develop in a fashion essentially comparable to that of plant cells. First there appeared a nucleus and then around this the new cell formed. In plants, the new nuclei appeared *within* the walls of a parent cell, but in animal tissues the nuclei first became manifest *outside* any of the old cells. The generation of cells "takes place in a fluid, or in a structureless substance in both cases. We will name this substance in which the cells are formed, cell-germinating material (Zellenkeimstoff), or cytoblastema. It may be figuratively, but only figuratively, compared to the mother-lye from which crystals are deposited."[16]

Here are the two crucial features for understanding the later theories and disputes about pulmonary consumption. We must keep in mind the concept of a mother liquor or blastema, which in plants occurred within rigid cell walls but in animal tissues was free-lying. Within this mother liquor the process of cellular development involved the appearance of a nucleus followed by the deposition of plasmatic substance.

*Cellular Tissue*

In the 18th and 19th centuries, anatomists, physiologists, and pathologists made frequent use of the term "cellular tissue." This, obviously, means a tissue characterized by cells. And, while that is precisely what the term does mean, there has arisen a vast confusion. The word "cellular," in this phrase, has Hooke's original meaning, namely, a porous structure more or less resembling a honeycomb. *Cellular tissue meant the loose connective tissue, composed of delicate fibrils separated by abundant tissue spaces* that might readily get distended with fluid or even with air.

This cellular tissue was widely distributed—e.g., in the deeper layers of the skin, or underlying the mucous membranes, or separating the various organs. The modern term is "areolar tissue," a phrase that stresses the spaces or interstices, and offers a contrast to the dense connective tissue such as tendon or fascia.

"Cellular tissue" had no relation whatever to the cells of Schleiden and Schwann. Great confusion resulted when writers used cellular tissue in its original sense and also talked about the cells as described by Schwann. In a single sentence, writers might mention the cells in the cellular tissue—the modern equivalent would be, cells in the loose connective tissue. Many otherwise excellent historians have failed to distinguish properly between "cell" as a biological unit and "cellular" as a particular form of connective tissue. I must exhort my readers to avoid the confusion.

### Blastema, Organization, and Vitality

Since cells were alleged to arise from the blastema, we may fairly ask, "What was the nature of this substance?" The answer stemmed from concepts that had their roots in both physiology and pathology.

Physiologists knew that the blood, circulating throughout the entire body, furnished all the material needed for nourishment, growth, and secretion. Especially important here is the concept of secretion, which at that time meant not merely a glandular product like saliva or bile, but also the subtle transudation of fluid whereby "an albuminous matter, in the state of liquid or of vapour, is constantly produced in every part of the system."[17] It comprises the moisture observed on every serous membrane, in the cellular tissue, and wherever an organ presents a surface. This form of secretion was sometimes called "a transpiration," or sometimes a "perspirable matter," meaning not the ordinary perspiration or sweat, but the "internal perspiration" of which we are not aware. This perspirable matter—secretion in its very broad sense—arose from the blood. Secretion was thus a halfway house between blood and solid tissues.

In the relations between the blood and the tissues, the study of coagulation was quite important. Physicians knew that blood, when flowing in the vascular channels, normally remained fluid, but outside the body it produced a clot. Responsible for the clot was a substance called "fibrin." Why, if fibrin existed within the circulating blood, clotting did not occur within the normal body, was not known. The absence of intravascular clotting was attributed to a "vital" property of the blood.

According to John Hunter a form of coagulation did take place within the living healthy body: through nutrition the fluid blood became transformed into solid tissue. In 1793 Hunter declared, "For as all the solid parts of the body are formed from the blood, this could not take place, if there did not exist in it the power of coagulating." Hunter went on to say that this property did not belong to the whole mass of circulating blood, but only to one component thereof, the "coagulating lymph." This represented, in a sense, the rough equivalent of the circulating fibrin, that is, the material that under certain circumstances formed a solid clot, and presumably was operative in the formulation of the solid tissues.[18]

The relations of the circulating blood and the solid tissues were obviously quite complex, but the chemists were able to provide some more or less relevant information. Physiologists recognized that the chemical composition of the blood did not differ essentially from that of the solids. Clearly, material seemed to pass out of the blood to become incorporated in a solid tissue, since their respective composition, as determined by the available chemical techniques, was similar.

Pathology was able to bring some added light. In disease, secretory activity showed alterations from the normal and, said Andral, "is liable to have its qualities considerably modified, so that in place of the fluid which should constitute its natural product, another substance may be found, differing from it in a greater or less degree." This new material, altered in quality from the normal, was called a "morbid secretion," that replaced the "natural perspiratory fluid."[19]

Morbid secretion served as a major concept to explain disease. Andral's text holds particular interest, for when it was published microscopic study had not contributed much to pathology, yet held out promise for the future. Andral's theories, propounded during this larval period of microscopy, furnished an excellent background for the data and theories of the 1840s.

Morbid secretions, studied by the pathologist, were highly variable, and offered great difficulty in classification, since no precise criteria were at hand. Andral, relying principally on gross observation, divided the new formations into two major groups: those which showed "no trace of organization or of vitality" and those which did show at least traces of "organization" and "vital action." In the first group the important examples were pus and tubercle; under the second heading he included fibrin from the blood and also the lesions we identify as cancer. (A third group, which comprised animal parasites, need not be considered here.)[20]

Today, in pathology, the term "organization" means the replacement of fibrin by connective tissue, through the activity of leucocytes, fibroblasts, macrophages, and endothelial sprouts. In the early part of the last century, however, this was not the case. The term meant, quite literally, having the properties of a bodily organ, that is, the characteristics of a living being (in contrast to the inert substances that the chemists dealt with). A morbid secretion became "organized" when it developed a nutrition of its own, was capable of reacting to various irritations and of having its own secretions and transudations. All these properties indicated vitality, which happened to correlate with the presence of blood supply. The blood was considered to be alive, and the presence of circulating blood meant that there was life in a secretion, which otherwise would be more or less a foreign body.

After the work of Schwann and the beginning of cell theory, however, a new criterion for organization arose, namely, the presence of cells, or their components. *A morbid secretion (or blastema) would show organization if it gave rise to cells or nuclei.* This indicated vitality, for inert chemical substances could not form cells. Some secretions might exhibit a high degree of organization, which meant that they not only gave rise to abundant cells but in addition would acquire a blood supply. Secretions that had a low degree of organization gave rise to few cells, and furthermore would not develop the other properties of vital tissues, such as the reaction to irritation. The presence of cells became the primary criterion of vitality, although the development of a blood supply was not ignored.

The theory of blastema that dominated pathology derived, as we have seen, from physiology, especially the study of secretion and the passage of fluid from the blood vessels into the tissues. Historians like to speak of this trend as "humoralism," by which they meant a dependence of disease on the fluid components of the body. This is sometimes a term of derision, but actually the doctrine of blastema, in the middle decades of the 19th century, was a superb synthesis of the latest scientific research and an intellectual construct excellently adaptive to the knowledge of the era.

*Scrofula*

Pulmonary consumption, as we have seen, was long recognized as a clinical entity whose defining features might vary according to the physicians who wrote about it. The important clinical signs were emaciation and wasting, cough, with the production of "pus," and fever of the particular type known as hectic.

When we try to understand the growth of knowledge about tuberculosis, we find that scrofula holds an interesting position. Of ancient lineage, it had several different names: struma, King's evil, écrouelle, and, in horses, farcy. The clinical features on which the diagnosis rested were the chronic swelling of lymph glands, principally in the neck, but the swellings might also affect the axilla, the groin, the mesentery, and other concealed parts of the body. Commonly there were complicating lesions, such as ulcerations of the skin and mucous membranes, with draining sinuses; and involvement of bones, joints, and soft tissues. Usually but not always the disease attacked children. It did not ordinarily produce emaciation, cough, or fever. The clinical features of scrofula were generally quite distinct from those of consumption.

The ulcerations in scrofula, usually related to the enlarged glands, formed a prominent part of the clinical picture. Describing these ulcers, Cullen declared: "Some heal up, while other tumours and ulcers appear in the vicinity. . . . In this way the disease goes on for several years; but very commonly in four or five years is spontaneously cured, the former ulcers being healed up, and no new tumours appearing." But sometimes there was a more unfavorable course, and he noted that patients who die of the disease often showed tubercles in the lung. Cullen, however, in his nosology, did not relate scrofula to consumption but thought there were similarities to syphilis.[21]

The occurrence of chronically swollen lymph glands, often with ulcers, with a more or less characteristic age distribution and course, does suggest a clinical unity, despite variation in such features as location of glands, degree of surface ulcerations, or involvement of bones and joints. The typical picture differed markedly from pulmonary consumption. Sometimes the two conditions occurred in the same patient, sometimes not. Some physicians believed in a close relation between scrofula and consumption; others denied the relationship. The vast literature, pro and con, I will not discuss in detail.

In the publications of this era the physicians generally assumed that scrofula, as observed clinically, was a single disease. Only later did they realize that what was called scrofula might actually comprise a number of quite distinct conditions, the most important of which was tuberculosis, while other diseases having nothing to do with tuberculosis might give symptoms comparable to scrofula. As we shall see, Villemin, in the 1860s made this abundantly clear, but in the 1840s and 1850s clinical and pathological discrimination was not yet sufficiently sharp to distinguish clearly between scrofula and tuberculosis.

*New Viewspoints from Microscopy*

Microscopy led to a massive accumulation of new data, but these gave rise to varying interpretations. Out of the difference of opinion new theories emerged that again led to what our present-day journalists would call a breakthrough. The story is quite dramatic, but I can pay special attention to only a few aspects. I will consider the validity of the blastema theory, its replacement by the modern cellular theory, the nature of the tubercle, the nature of caseation, the relationship of scrofula to tuberculosis, and the concept of tuberculosis as a disease entity.

In the 1840s Schwann exerted a marked influence. He had made important steps in establishing a nomenclature, emphasizing granules, nuclei, cells, and blastema. The nuclei, he thought, might exist as naked structures, or as formative agents that could go on to form complete cells. According to his views, granules, nuclei, and cells all derived from the blastema.

The pathologists of the mid-19th century studied many different diseases and encountered a wide range of structures. Receiving special attention were the formation of pus, of tubercle, and of cancer. These three were related in an important sense— they were all considered to be products of secretion, arising from separate blastemas that, in turn, derived from the blood. They were all considered examples of "new formations."

Pus, as a fluid substance, was relatively easy to examine. It contained abundant corpuscles, most of which had nuclei that seemed to divide and multiply. Although the pus corpuscles resembled in many ways the white corpuscles that circulated in the bloodstream, most observers believed that pus cells arose from a blastema that was deposited in the tissues.[22]

Microscopic study of tuberculous material showed many distinct features: fine granules, sometimes called molecules; an amorphous or flocculent material, later known as caseation, considered to be a coagulated protein; oval corpuscles or bodies that contained granules and might or might not have a nucleus. Other descriptions included naked nuclei, cells with distinct nuclei, and cells with multiple nuclei.

Before going further into the pathology of tuberculosis, I must clarify the nomenclature. The word tuberculosis, referring to a disease, derived from the old term "tubercle." This originally meant an anatomical structure, a small nodule or tumor, but this usage gradually became confined to the small structures found, e.g., in pulmonary consumption. These, in their great variety, had been excellently described by Bayle, Laennec, and others, who relied on gross observation only.

Further studies, especially with the microscope, paid special attention to the granular substance of cheesy appearance, found in consumption. This matter, at first called "tuberculous matter," might appear in minute amounts in the center of a barely visible tubercle, or it might exist in massive quantities in lungs of lymph nodes. It seemed to be something more or less characteristic, especially associated with the clinical disease that soon came to be known as tuberculosis. Whether this special substance was uniquely related to the disease was a moot point. But at any rate, the term "tubercle" acquired a dual meaning—the discrete small nodule and also the granular caseous matter. When the caseous substance was in question, the word "tubercle" was used in a generic sense, without any qualifying article. When, however, a discrete nodule was in question, pathologists spoke of "a" or "the" tubercle or, as with Virchow, a "true" tubercle. But "tubercle," unqualified, usually referred to caseous material as a general class.

This distinction, as we shall see, became especially significant with the work of Virchow. However, before we deal with this, we must further elaborate on the blastema theory.

Tubercle—caseous matter—was especially important in blastema theory, which, as we have seen, held that plasmatic material passed from the blood into the tissues and, once there, gave rise to cells. The blastemas, as a deposit or exudate, had varying potentialities to produce cells. There were three major types of exudate: inflammatory, cancerous, and tuberculous. Once these entered the tissues, they realized their different potentialities, one type producing pus, another cancer, and the third tubercle.

The caseous material was not the raw blastema but was rather the "first elaboration." We might say that the blood gave rise to the blastema, which in turn gave rise to tubercle. Why one blastema should produce pus with its abundant cells, another blastema give rise to cancer with equally abundant cells, and a third to tubercle, with very few cells, no one knew. The theorists could only fall back "on the inherent composition or constitution of the exudation itself."[23]

The different blastemas, then, each had its own intrinsic formative power, giving rise to greater or less numbers of cells of different character. On microscopic examination the morbid deposits of tubercle showed relatively few cells, but a great deal of granular matter that was not organized. Hence, tubercle, in contrast to suppuration or cancer, had relatively little "formative power."

The proponents of the blastema theory held that the nature of the exudation depended on the character and composition of the blood. If we seek more precise causes, we must study whatever factors "operate on the composition" of the blood to change it from a normal fluid to an abnormal one. Bennett,[23] for example, felt that in cancer, with its high degree of cellularity and organization, the blood contained an excess of nutritive material, while in tubercle the blood had a deficiency of nutritive material (in line with its low degree of organization). These speculative inferences reveal one trend of the blastema theory.

Another trend we can see in examining the relationships between tuberculosis and scrofula. Ancell, in 1852, gave some interesting sidelights. He belonged to the group that regarded scrofula as a form of tuberculosis, even though there was no conclusive evidence. For him tuberculosis was a general disease of the blood that could have local manifestations and varieties. The newer pathological anatomy, he said, had clearly shown that the various forms had a common origin. This origin, he believed, lay in the blood; tuberculosis "is strictly an idiopathic disease of the blood." But, since this fluid is very complex, the morbid constituents may differ and then give rise to different manifestations.[24]

Phthisis was the most important manifestation of tuberculosis. Scrofula, on the other hand, was a poorly defined term that indicated a local lesion elsewhere than in the lungs. Ancell believed "that there is one definite, although at present not strictly definable, constitution of the blood, upon which all the manifestations of tuberculous disease depend; and . . . that in both, 'scrofulosis' and 'tuberculosis,' they depend upon the same causes." Ancell did not say that the pathology and clinical course were identical in these two diseases, or even closely similar, but only that "as a whole, it is the same predisposition which tends to both scrofula and tubercle." The "local products" of both have "the same anatomical elements, and there are many strict analogies in their chemical composition," and both show the same reactions of softening.[25]

## The Contributions of Virchow

Improved technology and more precise observation sapped the foundation of the blastema theory until it collapsed in the 1850s. Its tenets proved indefensible in the light of new data and more logical inference. The principal credit for the overthrow of the blastema theory belongs to Rudolph Virchow (1821-1902), who contributed enormously to the progress of pathology. But he also severely muddled the concepts of tuberculosis until the confusion he introduced was resolved through the abilities of men like Jean-Antoine Villemin and Robert Koch.

Virchow began the study of pathology at a favorable time, when improved lenses were becoming available and when microscopy was emerging as a major discipline. He became thoroughly expert in a way that older pathologists like Rokitansky (1804-1878), raised in an earlier tradition, could never achieve. But unfortunately Virchow was dogmatic and arrogant—the other person was always wrong—and he leaped to many wrong conclusions.

Two interrelated principles underlay Virchow's mature doctrines. After first embracing the blastema theory, he soon changed his mind and denied the existence of any exudation that could give rise to new cells. But if new formations did not arise from any exudative mother-liquor, he had to account for their origin. Here he enunciated his second basic principle: that all cells arose from other preexisting cells, a doctrine summarized in the now familiar expression, *Omnis cellula e cellula*, a major concept in the expansion of biology and medicine.[26]

New-formed cells, claimed Virchow, were of two sorts. Cells that resembled existing tissue elements were called homologous and these arose directly from the precursors to which they were similar. But other new formations—such as pus, tubercle, and cancer—differed markedly from any normal tissue and their cells were called "heterologous." If there were no blastema to serve as a source, and if they were not obviously similar to normal constituents, their origin required explanation. Said Virchow, heterologous cells arose chiefly from cells of the connective tissue, which was very widely distributed throughout the body and comprised a widely dispersed source. In a functional sense the connective tissue replaced the blastema as the source of cells in new formations.

These pronouncements required considerable elaboration to carry any conviction. Much of the evidence was highly speculative and some represented a begging of the question. Even superficial observation showed that heterologous cells usually had little resemblance to normal connective tissue elements. Virchow solved this difficulty by pointing to "transitional" cell forms. Furthermore, we know from embryology that undifferentiated or young cells can develop in any of several directions. Hence the young connective tissue might give rise to a variety of new forms, different from the parent cells.

Virchow did not limit the source of new formations to the connective tissue—he thought, for example, that pus might also derive from transformed epithelial cells—but he denied that cells found in the tissues arose from the blood. This savored too much of the hated blastema theory. However much pus cells might resemble colorless corpuscles of the blood, they nevertheless had a *local tissue origin*.

Almost single-handed Virchow created the science that we call "general pathology." This studies not particular diseases like glomerulonephritis or typhoid fever but rather describes abnormal processes, bodily reactions that might occur in a variety of conditions and that are not themselves specific to any one disease. The various reactions of general pathology—such as atrophy, hypertrophy, inflammation, embolism, necrosis, fibrosis, calcification, fatty metamorphosis, and the like—are, so to speak, the vocabulary for understanding disease, terms that can appear in different combinations. The individual changes are not diagnostic.

Virchow paid special attention to these tissue reactions. However, his concern with general pathology induced a severe disregard of *diseases*. He was not in any sense a clinician. He did not deal with patients and his concern with tissue reaction, admirable in a limited sense, carried him into an extreme disregard of clinical evidence.

This attitude, as an intellectual trend, was made worse by what I can regard only as emotional overtones directed against French investigators like Bayle and Laennec. These men combined clinical acumen with autopsy studies to create a firm foundation for the understanding of tuberculosis. Virchow venomously rejected their claims and frequently made snide and gratuitous comments about their work. The French had joined clinical experience to pathological analysis. Virchow, with no clinical experience, devoted himself principally to the study of tissue reactions and denied the reality of the disease entity.

Of the various reaction patterns observable in tuberculosis, caseation is perhaps the most striking. Virchow devoted special attention to this topic and, in a way, this formed the focus for his ideas.

By the 1840s, in tuberculosis the opaque granular cheesy substance was thoroughly familiar to all investigators. It was variously known as caseous material, tuberculous matter, or simply as tubercle. The first two names suggest relation to the clinical disease, while the third carried overtones of the blastema theory. Whatever the name, the substance was well known but its essential nature was still obscure.

Today we know that this material, in tuberculosis, results from an antigen-antibody reaction, which produces a peculiar necrosis that usually is easily recognized in routine tissue sections. The amount and character of the caseation will vary according to the immunological status of the patient, the strain of the infecting bacillus, and the course of the disease. Sometimes this necrotizing process involves large areas of tissue, sometimes only a minute amount.

Virchow knew nothing of antigens and antibodies and their

interactions. He was contending mainly against the prevailing blastema theory, according to which the blood deposited in the tissues various cell-free materials that had the power of cell-formation. Those blastemas which produced suppuration or cancer had a strong cell-forming power, while the deposit responsible for tubercle had only a weak power. Hence tubercle—the immediate product of the blastema—was cell-poor. This tuberculous matter, which we are now calling caseation, had been regarded as an early stage in the disease process.

Virchow regarded this view, in his mature years, as colossal error. He showed that in tuberculosis the asserted relationship between caseation and cells should be reversed. The cells came first, arising from other cells pre-existing in the tissues and not from any exudation from the blood. Only when the cells underwent degeneration did the caseation—the tuberculous matter—come into being. If the caseous substance contained only a few cells, this meant that necrosis was virtually complete, and not, as the blastema theory would have said, that cell formation was in an early stage.

This interpretation of tuberculous matter as an end stage rather than an early production represents a profound advance in our knowledge, an advance for which Virchow deserves great credit. But in reaching this conclusion he had meanwhile gone severely astray. The early French investigators who had combined great clinical experience with their pathological studies appreciated the intimate relationship between clinical tuberculosis and the caseous matter, which they regarded as characteristic of the disease. Their clinical acumen and their skill in gross pathology were, however, hampered by faulty theory. Virchow, while he eventually corrected the theory, fell into a different error. He regarded caseation as an entirely non-specific reaction that, while it did occur in consumption, occurred also in cancer and in "ordinary" suppuration, and was by no means characteristic of anything.

Now, errors of fact are not of themselves especially important, for science travels along a highway built from previous mistakes. But Virchow's errors unfortunately were enormously influential. We can profitably study some of the steps by which he arrived at his conclusions.

Virchow based his doctrine on some early observations. In 1847, when he still had not repudiated the blastema theory, he published an important paper on cancer. Within a tumor he noted areas of cancer cells that showed "fatty metamorphosis." He also saw areas of "so-called tubercle-like masses," an observation that, he pointed out, Lebert had already recorded in 1844. Virchow described the appearances. In cancer the tubercle-like masses have "a great similarity to crude tubercle: they exhibit an opaque, yellowish white, friable substance, interspersed in different sized areas in the cancer." These, he thought, differed from ordinary "softening" (i.e., necrosis) through their "pulpy crumbly character." To this gross description he added only relatively brief microscopic description.[27]

In this early paper Virchow claimed to have seen the same change in liver cells and, more especially, in "pus cells." And here, "just as in cancer, it has given occasion for repeated confusion with tubercle [i.e., caseation]." As examples of tubercle-like changes in "pus," he pointed to the caseous masses found in bone and adjacent soft tissues that we now know are tuberculous in origin.

In various publications he described the steps by which necrosis took place. The cells get crowded together, fluid is resorbed, the cellular elements become shrivelled and lose their individuality, nuclei shrink, cell contents grow indistinct, fatty metamorphosis may occur, the cells turn into a crumbly granular mass wherein only fragments might be recognizable. The descriptions varied somewhat in different publications, but the unity of the process is clear. Under whatever conditions this sequence took place, the end result was caseation, a process nonspecific, even though present in tuberculosis. Indeed, "tuberculosis" was taking on the meaning of a histological sequence rather than a disease.

In all his subsequent papers Virchow continued to rely uncritically on his early observations. Caseation for him represented a cellular transformation that could be found in different and quite distinct conditions, namely, cancer and suppuration. In all three the end-result was the same reaction. From this it followed that "tubercle" (i.e., caseation) was not in any way characteristic of any disease (let alone serving as a diagnostic criterion, which some authors had suggested).

In subsequent papers Virchow sharpened the nomenclature. He spoke of tubercle-like metamorphosis, thus emphasizing the notion of change; then he used the term "tuberculization," and then, as the most precise designation, he spoke of "caseous metamorphosis," meaning thereby the process by which initially well formed cells underwent a series of changes, to end in a cheese-like mass. Caseation was "coordinate" with other types of tissue change, such as waxy or fatty or atheromatous degeneration.[28]

Virchow brought to a focus his doctrines of caseation in his discussions of scrofula, which, as we have seen, has to do especially with the lymph nodes. These, Virchow pointed out, readily enlarge. This reactive swelling occurs more readily in some people than in others. Such persons, he said, had a "lymphatic constitution" or constitutional predisposition, and show unusually severe swellings in response to rather trivial irritants that in other persons, or under ordinary circumstances, would arouse no reaction at all. He called this disproportionate reaction a "vulnerability." In susceptible persons swellings of the neck, for example, appear far more readily than in the normal and last for a long time, persisting even when the surface irritation has gone away. This special reactivity he attributed to a local "weakness" of the parts, and in scrofula the glands of the neck are especially affected. If a more general weakness occurs, then the lymph glands of the thorax and abdomen can also be involved.

According to Virchow the disease scrofula resulted from the aggregation of several factors. There was the predisposition—a constitutional inclination—and a local "weakness"; and there was an irritation that produced cellular proliferation. The local weakness of the "mother tissue" was carried over to these new-formed cells, products of the irritation. *Because of the weakness of the mother tissue*, the individual cells showed increased fragility, went to pieces quite readily, and developed early necrosis and caseation. This process affected not only the new-formed cells but also the original substance of the gland. The same type of change might also affect the various mucous membranes and the skin. The caseation was not specific to scrofula but was found in suppuration, in typhoid aggregates, in cancer, and "in many other new formations that are rich in cells."[29]

This necrotizing process might especially affect pus cells. Irritative reactions like catarrh and pustular exanthems could produce pus that might stagnate and then, like the hyperplastic cells of the lymph nodes, become thickened and caseous. A key point in Virchow's doctrine was this "tuberculization" of pus, the transformation of real pus into a caseous mass. This, he said, often occurred in scrofulous individuals. In proof, he pointed to the "caries" of bones, which he called "osteomyelitis suppurativa," an emphasis on pus formation. This lesion destroyed bone, led clinically to hunchback, and also to the accumulation of caseous matter in the soft tissue, known as cold abscesses. We know now that this material he called pus has no relation to real pus but represents a tuberculous reaction from the very beginning.

Virchow believed strongly that caseation was a non-specific tissue reaction that, since it occurred in a variety of non-related conditions, could have no special relationship to any single disease. The French investigators, on the other hand, had constantly emphasized the special relationship between caseation and tuberculosis. This view Virchow opposed, and in proof he claimed that he demonstrated caseation in cancer, suppuration, and other disorders. But for his examples of suppuration he selected lesions in bones and soft tissues, lesions that we now know are tuberculous in origin. Thus, Virchow was using tuberculous lesions to "prove" that caseation had no special relation to tuberculosis.

The modern reader must wonder why a pathologist of Virchow's abilities and stature should have gone so far astray. His errors were finally exposed through the brilliant work of Villemin and of Koch, who initiated a new era in the study of tuberculosis, concerned with progress in bacteriology.

## The Bacteriological Era

*Jean-Antoine Villemin*

Jean-Antoine Villemin (1827-1892) was one of the truly great investigators of tuberculosis. While he had sound knowledge of gross and microscopic pathology—indeed, some of his microscopic descriptions of tissue changes are unsurpassed—he never ceased to be a clinician, with a clinician's outlook. He carefully picked his way through the jungle of conflicting and often inadequate evidence, reasoned clearly and cogently, and performed critical experiments to prove his points. With his clear insight he made enormous progress in solving the problems of the day.

Villemin published various studies during the 1860s and his major contributions appeared in book form in 1868.[30] We should remember that one of Virchow's most influential papers, with extensive summaries of earlier views, appeared in 1865. Villemin, although he wrote in the shadow of Virchow's authority, showed the way to a new and fruitful approach. If we analyze the reasons for his success, we must lay special stress on his continuous clinical orientation. He was always concerned with the patient and with the disease entity.

In the best tradition of French medicine, the tradition that produced Bayle and Laennec, Villemin never lost sight of tuberculosis as a clinical phenomenon that pathology alone could not explain completely. Pathological findings required correlation with clinical information. Furthermore, he not only drew upon clinical and anatomical aspects of tuberculosis but he also attended to other diseases that might have some analogy with tuberculosis. With what we might call a global outlook, he took into account factors to which others had paid little attention, and perceived significance and inner connections that others had ignored.

Reasoning by analogy, Villemin was convinced that tuberculosis was a specific disease resulting from a specific infectious agent. In smallpox, for example, each individual lesion contained a "morbific matter" that could spread the disease. So too with glanders, which was also transmissible. He pointed to other diseases—such as typhoid fever, typhus, plague, yellow fever, swamp fever—for which a transmissible substance had not yet been so clearly implicated but which, by analogy suggested a specific agent that spread within the body. Such a hypothetical causal agent he designated as "virus," which, of course, must be understood not in the technical sense the word enjoys today but in its earlier sense of "poison"—an agency that produced an effect and that had specificity.

The disease tuberculosis, Villemin declared, shows a multitude of lesions, each of which must result from the direct action of the responsible agent carried into all the organs in an extremely fine state of division. He claimed that in its action the "cause" of tuberculosis bore the most strict analogy to the virus of smallpox or glanders.

Again and again Villemin returned to the question of specificity and to the inferences to be drawn from analogy. And when he emphasized the notion of a specific cause he was at the same time (and automatically) rejecting the concept of non-specific causes. The multiplicity of similar lesions rendered entirely unreasonable any belief that non-specific factors, such as cold or heat, or ordinary banal irritants, could produce tubercle. The only reasonable explanation was a specific agent. The cause of tuberculosis, he said, must be some substance spread throughout the organism, disseminated and transported by the *milieu intérieure*.[31]

Early physicians like Morton or Cullen lacked any concept of specificity but based their recognition of consumption on essentially clinical grounds. The great French investigators of the early 19th century emphasized the clinicopathological changes that underlay the clinical findings. Microscopy permitted finer analysis and discrimination, and led to hopes of finding specificity. Lebert[32] had suggested specific cells that he thought were uniquely diagnostic of tuberculosis, and, when this criterion failed, considerable attention was paid to caseation as perhaps the characteristic feature, the specific criterion.

Virchow claimed that caseation was a process entirely non-specific, the end result of many different pathological progressions and origins. Villemin, although not a disciple of Virchow, agreed that caseation was not a sound diagnostic criterion. He emphasized the drawbacks of microscopic study and concluded that there was no distinctive pathological criterion that by itself could identify that disease. Caseation would not serve, and neither would the anatomical tubercle. The tubercle alone was not specific, regardless of whether we look at the cell components, their configuration, their origin, or their progressive changes (metamorphoses). The same type of cells and the same changes can be found in other diseases entirely distinct from tuberculosis.

Villemin discussed particularly syphilis and glanders. These diseases are ordinarily distinguishable pathologically from tuberculosis, yet the fine shades of difference "would be inadequate to dispel *all uncertainty, if we relied only on the histological appearance.*" He is saying that microscopic discrimination does not have complete validity. For identification the physician must depend not on single differentiating features but on an ensemble of factors. Speaking of identifying features, Villemin said, "In the present state of our knowledge we can find these only in the manner of distribution, the site, the diversity of the process, the dissemination in the body, in the progression and the appearance [*physionomie*] of the disease itself, but above all, in the *morbid cause.*" For identification we must thus rely on a congeries of factors, on patterns and combinations. Thus, granulomas in the lung with emaciation, night sweats, bronchitis, and the like pertained to tuberculosis, while different combinations were typical of glanders or syphilis. For ordinary practice these characteristics were adequate, and only in exceptional cases were they insufficient.[33]

For the most part, then, such approximations were adequate, but the scientist wants to achieve greater precision. Villemin made great progress through his conviction that certain diseases had specific infectious agents as their "cause." The clinical features were not specific, and neither (in any rigid sense) were the pathological findings. Specificity must lie in the cause, and by this he meant a discrete and unique infectious agent that determined the character of individual diseases.

He capitalized, so to speak, on certain resemblances between tuberculosis, syphilis, and glanders. The similarities in their pathology argued for a similarity in essential nature. He believed that syphilis and glanders each had specific etiological agents. These, to be sure, had not been isolated, but the two diseases were each capable of experimental transmission to other hosts.

For Villemin, tuberculosis, syphilis, and glanders had some sort of a family relationship. Then he reasoned that if the three diseases were similar in some of their pathological reactions, and if two of them were transmissible, experimentally, then the third should also be transmissible. And thus he justified, on the grounds of analogy, his experimental studies regarding the transmissibility of tuberculosis. His extensive experiments may seem to us relatively crude, but he abundantly proved his point.

First Villemin studied the natural occurrence of tuberculosis among various animal species and also tested out the susceptibility of animals to inoculation with matter taken from human cases. He indicated the similarities between the disease in cows and in humans, and determined that the rabbit was an especially good subject for transmission experiments. The occurrence of the natural disease in birds he could not establish with accuracy and he concluded that the answer remained problematical. Details of observations and experiments are oblique to our main interest.

Villemin's most important conclusions derived from his work on the rabbit, which proved to be the most satisfactory animal; in other species such as the dog, cat, sheep, and goat, the results were at best equivocal. He successfully reproduced tuberculosis in animals, using caseous material and tubercles taken from various sites in man. And he also successfully transmitted tuberculosis from the cow to the rabbit. In some experiments he made successful transfers from man to rabbit to a second rabbit. He also determined the infectious nature of sputum, bronchial secretions, and even blood.

The precise details of Villemin's experiments need not be recounted. Even with his limited experimental techniques, he proved that tuberculosis was an infectious disease that could be transmitted to susceptible hosts such as the rabbit; and that a wide range of material—different types of lesions as well as sputum and (sometimes) blood—could induce the experimental disease. He also proved the "identity" of the human disease and the naturally occurring disease in cattle.

Villemin greatly enlarged our knowledge and quite adequately established his contention: tuberculosis was a specific entity entirely comparable to syphilis or to smallpox, and a transmissible agent—a "virus"—could appropriately be considered the "cause." However, we must remember that he still did not have any truly sharp criterion for the diagnosis of tuberculosis. Especially in lower animals there could be equivocal lesions, difficult to interpret, that could give rise to uncertainty regarding the diagnosis.

Unfortunately Villemin could not provide any definitive solution to the relationship of scrofula to tuberculosis. His experiments did not furnish convincing data one way or the other. The term "scrofula" centered around swelling of lymph nodes, especially in the neck. Mere caseation of lymph nodes, insisted Villemin, was in itself non-specific. It could be found in a variety of conditions—e.g., in syphilis, glanders, and typhoid fever, which, by general consent, were accepted as discrete diseases. It was also to be found in tuberculosis, whose status remained a matter of dispute. And caseation was also found in other conditions that had nothing to do with any of these.

Villemin felt strongly that the caseous lymph nodes found in syphilis or glanders or typhoid must be excluded from the category of scrofula. What, then, is left? There remain cases manifestly associated with tuberculosis of the lungs, and those which are not. To what extent, then, must these two residues be kept distinct? As I interpret Villemin, scrofula would apply only to those caseous lymph nodes which remain after you subtracted all instances where a specific disease is involved. Scrofula, for him, is thus a non-specific condition.

Scrofula, Villemin insisted, had nothing in common with tuberculosis except the caseation, a property that was shared with syphilis, glanders, and typhoid fever. All these latter diseases,

however, had an "essential nature," while scrofula came into
being only as the result of diverse and non-specific factors—*sous
l'influence des déterminations les plus diverses et les plus banales.*
Instead of having discrete specific causes, as did tuberculosis,
the caseous lymph nodes in scrofula resulted from "banal" causes
or non-specific reactions.[34]

## Robert Koch

Villemin had conclusively established that tuberculosis was an
infectious disease. We can regard him as an explorer who, having climbed a mountain peak, could see the goal ahead but had
no way of getting there himself. Robert Koch (1843-1910), by
demonstrating the infectious agent and proving its relation to
the disease, reached that goal.

In 1868, when Villemin gathered together his various contributions and published them in book form, the "Golden Age"
of bacteriology was just beginning. Of all the scientists who
created that discipline, Koch was one of the most brilliant, yet,
of course, he built upon the foundations established by others.
A great many men had studied various aspects of infectious diseases and the agents that might possibly be implicated. Many
different lines of investigations converged—and gave rise to
many conflicts. Any selection of names would be utterly incomplete and therefore perhaps misleading, but I want to indicate
a few especially relevant figures. There was Agostino Bassi
(1773-1856), who carried on fundamental researches on diseases
of silk worms (that had great relevance, actually, to human disease); Jacob Henle (1809-1885), who enunciated clearly the
basic principles that must underlie our knowledge of infectious
diseases but whose work aroused relatively little contemporary
attention; Louis Pasteur (1822-1895), whose studies on spontaneous generation, fermentation, and silk-worm diseases had, by
the 1860s, exerted great influence on contemporary research;
and Joseph Lister (1827-1912), who, influenced by Pasteur's
work, studied putrefaction and sepsis and introduced a technique
for combatting sepsis through carbolic acid spray (1867).

Meanwhile microscopic examination of tissues and secretions

had shown abundant microorganisms of the most diverse kinds—fungi, bacteria, spirochetes, vibrios, trichinae and other metazoa. These "germs" were found in normal tissues and in disease states, and their role was a matter of dispute and speculation.[35] In the first two-thirds of the 19th century there was already a vast literature dealing with microorganisms, with many assertions and counter-assertions regarding their role. The so-called germ theory of disease had many roots.

Robert Koch, perhaps the greatest of the 19th-century microbiologists, was a man of fantastic energy and great clarity of thought. He did his early work under conditions of extreme difficulty. As district-health officer in a small community, he also engaged in private practice, and in whatever spare time he could find he conducted his experiments in a primitive laboratory that he established in his home. That he could accomplish so much, under such adverse conditions, is a testament to his genius.

His first great work was on anthrax, a disease that, despite considerable attention from other investigators, was poorly understood. Koch, in his own home-built laboratory, solved the major problems of pathogenesis when he demonstrated the existence of spores, and indicated their role in the disease and the relations of bacteria and host. Although hitherto completely unknown to the scientific world, he won instant recognition when he demonstrated his findings and procedures to Ferdinand Cohn, the leading bacteriologist of the time. Koch, after publishing this work in 1877, continued his researches with important studies on wound infections.

When we reflect on the reasons for Koch's achievements, we must appreciate not only his insight into the crucial aspects of a problem, but also his technical virtuosity and his ability to create procedures that served the needs of his research and enabled him to prove his ideas. He made fruitful innovations in staining methods, isolation techniques, and cultural media. These technical aspects were indispensable parts of his successes.

In 1880, through the efforts of highly placed friends, Koch finally received a full-time appointment in Berlin, where he could devote all his tremendous energies to research and could have reasonably adequate facilities. In 1881 he began his studies on tuberculosis: in August of that year he inoculated his first guinea pigs with the tissues of an ape that had contracted the spontaneous disease. By March of 1882 he had made such vast progress that he felt ready to present his first report. This paper, published on April 10, 1882, is one of the great masterpieces of medical literature. With technical elegance and clear insight he provided answers to the problems that had puzzled physicians for hundreds of years, and established standards of rigor, standards that Henle had previously indicated but had never brought to fruition.[36]

By the latter part of the 19th century the concept of an infectious disease carried the assumption that some "parasite" or infectious agent would somehow be demonstrable. There was also the vague expectation that finding such a parasite meant that the "cause" had been discovered. Such a view, however, lacked any cogency, and there was no way to convince anyone who was contrary-minded. And, in the budding science of pathology and bacteriology, contrary minds abounded.

In tuberculosis no one had been able to demonstrate bacteria with any degree of constancy. Koch at first was no more successful than anyone else, but his genius for investigation led him to devise a new staining technique that showed, with great regularity, rod-shaped bacteria of rather characteristic appearance. Armed with this powerful new weapon, by which he could identify bacteria, hitherto unstainable, he systematically investigated tuberculous tissues from a variety of sources, as well as cases of scrofula, whose tuberculous nature, we have seen, was by no means unequivocally established. In almost all material, drawn from human cases and from animals that had become spontaneously ill, Koch found the characteristic rods. And he also had at his disposal a vast number of animals that he had inoculated with tuberculous matter and that had succumbed to the disease. Here too, with complete regularity, he could demonstrate the bacteria in the tissues.

In his classic monograph Koch described in considerable detail the different kinds of tuberculosis that he examined and the tissues that he studied. He concluded the first part of his work with the assertion, "On the basis of numerous observations I consider it as proved that in all tuberculous diseases of man and animals, bacteria are present that I designate as tubercle bacilli, and that are distinguished from all other micro-organisms by their characteristic properties."[37]

However, this constant association did not prove that the bacilli stood in a causal relation to the disease, despite considerable probability for the assumption. Then Koch indicated the requirements before such a causal connection could be established. The proof involved the following steps. The bacterium must be recovered from the tissues, and propagated successively in artificial culture medium until all contaminating material had been removed. When this pure culture, free of all contamination, was injected back into an animal host, there must result the same disease picture that occurred when the crude material had been injected. If the bacteria in pure culture could produce the same disease as did the crude infectious material, then and then only could the bacteria be considered the "causal" agent responsible for the infectious property.

These requirements had never before been fulfilled for any human infectious disease. When we say that a disease is infectious, we merely state that *something* carries the disease from one case to another. But to specify what that something might be, and to establish the assertion beyond all reasonable doubt, was a challenge that had never before been met for a human disease. The difficulties in achieving such a rigorous proof were severe.

The tubercle bacillus would not grow on ordinary media that would support the growth of other organisms. Koch had to devise special media on which the bacilli would grow, and he had to create techniques for isolating the bacilli from any possible contaminants. After he had solved the technical problems, Koch fulfilled the requirements of his postulates in a remarkably concise fashion. He isolated the tubercle bacilli, propagated them in pure culture through several generations, and then, when he reinjected the bacteria back into appropriate animal hosts, reproduced the disease, exactly as it appeared when crude tuberculous matter had been used. He gave abundant details of his experiments that we do not need to repeat here.

Koch thus settled two major problems. He demonstrated that

the bacilli in the tuberculous tissue were the "cause"—he used this term in a rather simplistic sense, and we will discuss the topic at considerable length in Chapters 9 and 10. Then he showed that at last there was a sharp criterion for the diagnosis of the disease. Hitherto there was no definite way of making an assured diagnosis. Now, however, it would not be difficult to decide what was and what was not tuberculosis. The answer would derive not from any histological characteristic but from the demonstration of the tubercle bacillus. As a result of Koch's work, and with the criterion he established, miliary tuberculosis, caseous pneumonia, caseous bronchitis, intestinal and glandular tuberculosis, the disease *"Perlsucht"* in cattle, as well as spontaneous and inoculation tuberculosis in animals, are all identical. They were all many different forms of one disease.

However, the problem of scrofula Koch did not solve. His results with staining procedures and inoculation experiments were equivocal, and his experiments, he declared, were not sufficiently numerous to reach a decision. A large proportion of the cases were tuberculous, and perhaps all, but the problem had to remain unsettled.

While Koch brought answers to problems that had troubled physicians for many centuries, these solutions opened the door to a vast number of new questions that previously could not have received any sort of meaningful answer. All these new problems had to do with what we can call "pathogenesis." How do the different forms of the disease arise? What factors are responsible for the remarkably varied appearance that can occur in different cases? The answers involve not merely bacteriology and pathology, but also a new but closely related science, immunology. And with the study of immunology we enter the fifth phase of the history of tuberculosis.

## THE IMMUNOLOGICAL ERA

Koch's discovery seemed to solve the important problems connected with tuberculosis, but actually the solution of one problem served merely to emphasize a host of others. Clinically the disease had long been known to exhibit great variety. It could progress slowly or rapidly, remain relatively limited or spread widely. "Galloping consumption" and miliary tuberculosis contrasted with the slower forms. The disease could show remissions and exacerbations. It might seem cured, only to break out again many years after the patient thought himself well. Autopsies might disclose perhaps merely scattered tubercles, perhaps extensive pneumonic consolidation, perhaps destruction with cavitation, or perhaps negligible cavitation but considerable fibrosis. How to explain all these different forms?

Although such features were well recognized long before Koch made his great discovery, they had remained as bare data, to be accepted rather than explained, or, if explained, only through speculation. However, once the tubercle bacillus was identified, there seemed a likelihood that these problems could find solutions.

In the 1880s and early 1890s the question of cure or prevention also assumed some importance. Pasteur had successfully attenuated the microbes of anthrax and of chicken cholera and had already produced a remedy against the bite of the rabid animal. Koch wanted similar successes with tuberculosis. In the course of his work he discovered what we now call "tuberculin," an extract of the culture of the bacteria. He thought this would be curative for tuberculosis. The claims proved unfounded, and the clinical trials actually led to considerable harm. Koch's reputation, enormously high to begin with, suffered from this failure, especially since he persisted in claiming some therapeutic efficacy. However, with the therapeutic aspects we will not be further concerned.

The work rested on an important discovery known as Koch's phenomenon. Tubercle bacilli inoculated into a normal healthy guinea pig produced only a slow reaction. In a few weeks there would develop at the site of injection an indolent nodule that eventually ulcerated, and that persisted as the infection gradually spread and the animal succumbed. If, however, an animal already infected received a second inoculum the reaction was totally different. At the second site there appeared within a day or two a violent inflammatory reaction with necrosis and sloughing.

But this violent reaction went on to rapid healing of the site, contrasting markedly with the slow but inexorable progression of the first injection.

This altered reaction, known as hypersensitivity, could also be induced by an extract of broth culture. The extract contained no live bacteria but only the products of the bacteria. The substances responsible for the reaction, eventually subjected to searching chemical analysis, produced an effect only in animals exposed to tuberculosis but not in normal animals. The phenomenon, which led eventually to the tuberculin test, proved to be a major foundation for the larval science of immunology.[38]

In the 1880s and early 1890s bacteriology made tremendous strides as did the new and related science of immunology. The era saw many discoveries—numerous pathogenic bacteria, toxins separable from bacteria, antitoxins, antibodies, the role of cells in the defense mechanism, the serologic specificity of bacteria, special biological reactions related to bacterial products and blood fractions—all these and many more began to circumscribe the new sciences. I will not even mention the great names or specify the important discoveries. The reader should consult the standard histories of bacteriology and immunology.

The data of tuberculosis, as studied by ingenious investigators, seemed to center around certain concepts derived from observation and experiment. Although they may sound like mere verbalisms, they have a definite empirical and operational content.

1. Strains of tubercle bacilli differ in *virulence*. This means only that a measured quantity of bacilli of one strain can produce a greater or lesser reaction than would the same quantity of a different strain. The quality of virulence can be enhanced or diminished.

2. The *quantity* of the infectious agent plays a role in the clinical picture. For a given strain a large inoculum will produce a more intense effect than will a smaller inoculum.

3. Hosts differ in their *native resistance*. The rat, for example, is "by nature" more resistant to infection than is the rabbit.

Humans, although they cannot be studied experimentally, like rabbits and rats, nevertheless seem also to have varying degrees of native resistance to infection.

4. Humans as well as animals differ in the degree of *hypersensitivity* they exhibit, that is, the inflammatory reaction that may develop as a result of a previous exposure to the agent. This, of course, is an elaboration of the Koch phenomenon. Some patients develop a violent sensitivity to the products of the tubercle bacillus, with an intense inflammatory reaction and considerable necrosis; in others the reaction is mild. Hypersensitivity is responsible for the necrosis and resulting cavitation seen in some cases of tuberculosis but not in others.

5. *Acquired resistance* is a variable much more difficult to analyze. The concept involves the ability of the patient to overcome the infection once it has been initiated, in contrast to the power to resist an infection from the very beginning. To what extent these may be modifications of a single variable we cannot at present be sure. At issue are the complex reactions by which an infection is overcome. The relation of hypersensitivity to the processes of healing and resistance is moot.

These variables interact one with the other, and the interactions serve to explain the different clinical and pathological manifestations. Thus, for a given degree of native resistance, a strain of bacteria having a heightened virulence can induce infection that otherwise might not have taken place. A patient with a feeble reaction of hypersensitivity may show much less caseation and cavitation than would a patient with a high degree of hypersensitivity. And so too with the various permutations and combinations.

These concepts became more concrete as immunology developed into its present complexity. The physical chemistry of highly specific blood proteins, the complicated cytology and biochemistry of the reticulo-endothelial system, the relation of specific cells to particular immunological reactions, the sensitization and physico-chemical alteration of cells as a result of antigenic action, the interactions of cells through chemical mediators, the different kinds of hypersensitivity reactions and their correlations with different types of lymphocytes and specific protein moieties—these are some of the topics relevant to modern understanding of tuberculous infection.

The clinical disease depends on the presence of the bacillus, to be sure, but in the present immunological era greater importance rests on what the older physicians called the internal factors. These we now interpret as the multiple features that we lump together as the immunological status of the patient. These relate to the topics of susceptibility, resistance, and reactivity. And these, in turn, are affected by other factors. Long before there was any science of immunology, physicians recognized that consumption was more likely to occur at certain times, such as puberty, than at others; and that some infections, or other disease like diabetes, or other conditions like pregnancy, could affect the course of tuberculosis. Now, through the study of immunological and cytological factors, scientists can make fine correlations that were unthinkable a century ago.

However, two caveats are in order. Much of the new information in immunology is fragmentary and the concepts still in flux. Evidence derived from in vitro experiments is limited, beset with exceptions and discordances. Extrapolation of results takes us into areas where clinical relevance is suggestive but far from definitive. I am reminded of the overall situation that obtained in the 1840s, when investigators brought forward enormous quantities of observations that had to be sifted and their relevance determined. In immunology clarification and simplifications will eventually come, but they have not yet arrived.

In tuberculosis we can designate the present as the era of immunology, whereby the infection is being explained through immunological mechanisms. There are already portents of the next stage, which may prove to be the era of heredity, wherein perhaps hereditary factors will determine the immunological factors that will in turn determine the pathological picture and the clinical course.

In this brief survey of tuberculosis we can see a steady progression of information, a growth of new concepts, a broadening of explanatory factors, a progressive complexity, and new modes of discrimination that have become fabulously precise. In each era the best investigative minds immersed themselves in the problems appropriate for that stage, and floundered among difficulties that were resolved only in a succeeding stage. Each stage depended on improved insight, technology, and discrimination.

Each era was searching for enlightenment. In the early stages the searchers had, for illumination, only a candle, but gradually the mode of illumination increased massively. What were the investigators able to see in the available light? I suggest that through the centuries the acuity of vision was the same. The differences lay in the mode of illumination.

*SOME BASIC CONCEPTS*

———————<>◄ ►<>———————

## CHAPTER 3

# Signs and Symptoms

## I

*If we get away from any medical context* and consider terms in their popular or "ordinary" sense, there is nothing mysterious about a sign. Most people would think, perhaps, of a sign on the street corner, identifying the name of the street, or perhaps on the highway, telling us which exit to take. These are everyday usages of the word.

Let me ask a question, "When is a sign not a sign?" This is not an idle conundrum but a serious question whose answer has considerable import. Let me give the answer before offering any explanation. I maintain that a sign ceases to be a sign when you cannot read it. The *meaning* has disappeared and the alleged sign becomes only another corporeal object (or, in more technical terms, merely a phenomenon).

To indicate the problem involved, let me mention a personal incident. One winter's day I was driving on an unfamiliar freeway, with instructions to leave it at a given exit, marked, I had been told, by a particular sign. After an appropriate number of miles I could see in the distance what I assumed was the proper sign, but when I came close I found it completely coated with ice, and totally illegible. What I saw was still a rectangular object, erected at the side of the road. It looked as if it ought to be a sign, but it conveyed no message, no meaning. It was merely another indifferent object by the roadside.

The essence of a sign is to convey information. Two reasons might keep us from getting the message: a physical impediment (like ice) keeps the message from reaching our sensorium; or there may be a mental impediment, such as a failure to understand the markings, even though they do reach the sensorium.

As an instance, we need merely note the traveler in a foreign country whose language he does not understand. Such a traveler may pause, for example, before a public toilet, trying to decide whether the words on the door mean "men" or "women." For the common western languages this is only rarely troublesome, but in the Orient there can be great difficulty.

In ordinary speech the word "sign" may refer to a physical object—the wood or metal or plastic—on which the words or other symbols are placed. Yet in the strict sense the "sign" refers to the symbols that convey the message, so that the physical object is really the vehicle rather than the sign. If the symbols are physically obscured, or if we do not understand them, we still have the physical object, but it no longer conveys any meaning. To say, "This is a sign that I cannot read" confuses the two senses of the word. Ordinarily the confusion makes little practical difference, but the distinction will be important, as we shall see, when we discuss signs in medicine.

A sign must necessarily have, as a correlate, a "thing signified"; and that which it signifies, that to which it refers, represents its meaning. "Sign" and "thing signified" are inseparable, like the two sides of a coin, or the inside and the outside of a circle. To have a sign that does not signify anything is like having a coin with one side only. In his idle moments, the reader might try to visualize this.

## II

When we return to a medical context and ask the same questions, "What is a sign?" and "When is a sign not a sign?" we encounter great confusion. The medical context is so far removed from everyday usage that we seem to be using a different language. To be sure, most physicians would deny that any confusion existed and in proof they would point to a medical dictionary or to a standard text by recognized medical authorities. There we do indeed have simplicity, but the pat simplicity of the answers is, in my opinion, specious and anti-historical, stultifying to thought.

In medicine the term "sign" is intimately connected with the term "symptom."[1] Currently "signs and symptoms" tend to come out in a single breath, as a unit, rather than as two distinct terms. They have to do with disease and are crucial in reaching a diagnosis. But, while they go together like ham and eggs, they are also quite distinguishable. Stedman's dictionary offers straightforward definitions: a symptom is "any morbid phenomenon or departure from the normal in function, appearance, or sensation, experienced by the patient and indicative of disease." The crucial concepts here: the symptom is something abnormal, relevant to disease, and experienced by the patient. The patient may notice, say, a swelling that causes no pain or impairment of function; or, he may be aware of untoward sensation that may range from severe pain, as with a ureteral stone, to vague feelings of discomfort after meals; or he may become aware of impairment function, such as visual disturbance, or difficulty in performing rapid finger movements. According to the definition, all of these would represent symptoms.

If now we turn to "sign" we find the following definition. "Any abnormality indicative of disease, discoverable by the physician at his examination of the patient: a sign is an objective symptom of disease; a symptom is a subjective sign of disease." Symptoms and signs apparently differ in only a single feature, that the one is subjective and the other objective. "Objective" is not defined, but ordinary usage would seem to indicate, first, something not related to the consciousness of the patient, i.e., having a "physical" as opposed to a "mental" existence, and, second, something apparent to any competent observer.[2]

Innumerable other authors repeat these ideas. Thus, "A *symptom* is subjective sensation or other personal observation that the patient describes to the physician. A *sign* is an abnormality observed by the physician during his physical examination." Or again, "A patient consults his physician because of unpleasant or unusual subjective sensations (symptoms) that interfere with his comfort or productivity. . . . Signs are the objective evidence of an illness that the physician detects by physical examination." Repeatedly we find the correlations, symptoms—patients—subjectivity; and signs—physicians—objectivity.[3]

An important variant we sometimes find expressed by the

phrase that the physician "elicits" the signs of disease, whereas the patient "describes" his symptoms. One dictionary states specifically: "The term 'physical sign' is generally applied to symptoms of which the patient does not complain but which are elicited upon examination."[4] Here the subjectivity of the symptom does not seem to be critical or even essential. Important, however, is the special expertise or even special apparatus that may be necessary to discover a sign. The physician, thus, can use his special knowledge and his command of apparatus to bring forth various objective phenomena related to the illness. The patient, however, does not need either expertise or apparatus to complain of pain.

The layman or the beginning medical student who wants to keep things tidy can be quite puzzled by all this. How do signs *really* differ from symptoms? The subjective-objective distinction is rather nonsensical, for the patient may complain of some highly objective phenomena. If the patient tells his physician, "Doctor, I have a swelling in my arm-pit," is he talking about a sign or a symptom? Or is the swelling a symptom until the doctor confirms it, at which point it becomes a sign? Or is it a disease? And if the patient, pressing his chest, tells his wife, "I think I am having a heart attack," how much is symptom and how much is sign? Will we say that the pain in the chest and the prostration are symptoms, and the sweating, pallor, and thready pulse are signs?

And what happens when it is the physician himself who becomes ill? Will he take on the posture of Pooh-Bah, and divide himself up into his various capacities and functions: "As patient, I have the symptom of a sore throat, while, as physician I observe in the mirror the signs of redness and swelling of the pharynx. As a patient, I feel a tightness in my chest and have a cough, while as physician I note that the sputum is scanty and mucoid; as a patient I feel hot, and when, as a physician I want to elicit some signs, I find that my pulse is 95 and by taking my temperature, I find that the thermometer reads 101."

Perhaps it is not quite fair to make fun of all this and deliberately choose trivial examples. But the contrasts so far offered, between patient and physician, between subjective and objective, between manifested and elicited, are so utterly misleading, and yet so uncritically accepted, that a little ridicule is a good thing. If a formulation cannot exclude absurdities, it is, to say the least, not very rigorous. Indeed, the current definitions of signs and symptoms are so lacking in rigor that they constitute a travesty on science—and on what we fondly regard as scientific medicine.

These present-day views, however widely accepted, I regard as quite faulty, at variance not only with ordinary usage but with the entire history of medicine up to the past century. I want now to present the traditional view, and then in the next section I will show how this became perverted into the present usage.

The Galenic tradition is surprisingly useful—and sometimes indispensable—for understanding the problems of today. Galen had distinguished theoretical medicine from the practical. Theoretical knowledge was embodied in texts called *Institutes of Medicine*. These consisted of five segments: physiology, pathology, semiology, hygiene, and therapeutics. This subdivision remained important in medical writings through the 17th and much of the 18th centuries, and then, under the influence of specialization and the increased volume of knowledge, each component of the *Institutes* required texts in its own right. We will be concerned only with pathology.

Pathology, then as now, dealt with disease. The neogalenists—the 16th- and 17th-century authors who wrote in the Galenic tradition—divided pathology into three divisions that dealt respectively with the disease, its causes, and its symptoms. This division becomes intelligible if we think of symptoms not in the present-day sense but as manifestations. Early authors like Fernel or Sennert defined symptom as an *affectus praeter naturam*. *Affectus* comes from *ad* and *facere*, and had the sense of acting upon, and referred specifically to the way that the disease acted upon the patient. The *affectus* might refer to a state of the mind or of the body. The important feature was the relation to the disease. Fernel stressed *affectus praeter naturam ex morbo profec-*

*tus,*[5] a manifestation arising from a disease. The symptom was secondary to the disease. Disease and symptom were equally contrary to nature, but the primacy rested with the disease, while the symptom was secondary.

These older notions of pathology we can readily transpose to modern terminology. Present-day students are taught the manifestations of disease, i.e., the way the disease affects the patient. For example, in pneumonia there would be pain in the chest, fever, difficulty in respiration, cough, sputum of a special character. There would also be purely morphologic features such as exudation, consolidation, and so on, in ever-increasing detail. These are all *praeter naturam* and they follow (or some might say, constitute) the pneumonia. Galen had said that the symptoms "follow" the disease as a shadow follows the body.[6]

Older writers distinguished the different classes of symptoms, corresponding to the three subdivisions of pathology. There are symptoms that manifest diseases, others that manifest causes, and others that indicate other symptoms. It is a little startling for the modern reader to think of a symptom of a symptom, as distinct from a symptom of a cause or of a disease, but some examples will clarify the distinctions.

Thus, cough could be a symptom of a disease. It could occur in many different conditions, such as catarrh, consumption, or peripneumonia (modern lobar pneumonia). On the other hand, edema could be the symptom of a cause (such as plethora) but would not tell us what diseases might be relevant. *The symptom was that which was caused by something else.* Some pulmonary disease caused the cough, while the plethora (itself a cause, not a disease) caused the edema.

The "symptom of a symptom" can be clarified by a modern example. Fever is a symptom of many different diseases, and it manifests itself in many different ways, including a skin that is hot to the touch. The physician who places his hand on the forehead of a patient and finds that the skin is hot is thereby attending to a symptom of a symptom, that is, to a manifestation (or effect) caused by the fever (which is itself a symptom). Hence the physician perceived the symptom of a symptom.

We may now ask, "What about signs in relation to disease?"

The older physicians had clear notions on the nature and functions of signs, but expressed their ideas in rather unfamiliar language. Signs are the marks, the *indicia*, that pointed to diseases, the information that permits us to work backward from the effect to the cause. This will be quite obvious if we think of diseases situated within the body and thus not amenable to direct observation. These could be known only through inference.

Let the older physicians speak for themselves. In the 16th century Jean Fernel wrote: "Diseases hidden in the innermost recesses of the body, that cannot be distinguished or perceived through the senses, are understood only by signs. With these as evidence [*rerum indiciis*] the mind is led by sound reasoning [*recta ratione*] to penetrate into what is hidden, and expose to view whatever is wrapped in obscurity; and [the mind] seems to perceive them visually [*oculis*]."[7]

Daniel Sennert, in the 17th century, declared: "By the term *signs* are to be understood all those things that indicate something else [*rem aliquam significant*]; or, all evidence that discloses [*patefaciunt*] something unknown and hidden." And early in the 18th century Antoine Deidier defined sign as "anything which, when known, leads to the further knowledge of something else that was unknown."[8]

Signs get transmuted into knowledge not by direct sensory perception but by a process of reasoning. For Boerhaave, in the early 18th century, the term "signs" applied to those phenomena "which, known by the senses, demonstrate through proper reasoning the presence, nature, condition, or outcome, whether of health or of disease and death."[9]

I will offer only one other example, from a text of 1813. For August-Jacques Landré-Beauvais a sign is "every phenomenon, every symptom, by means of which we can attain knowledge of hidden effects." Then he phrased very clearly the essential feature: "A sign, essentially, is a conclusion that the mind draws from the symptoms apparent to the senses [*observés par les sens*] while a symptom is only a matter of sense perception [*n'est qu'une perception des sens*]. Signs pertain to judgment, and symptoms to the senses."[10]

The import of all this is clear. Signs, by pointing to something beyond themselves, involve inference. A symptom—a phenomenon relevant to health—becomes a sign when to it we apply reasoning and judgment, and reach a conclusion not present in the original perception. A symptom is a phenomenon that we observe without attaching any specific meaning to it.

Essential here is the distinction between perception (or experience) and reason (between what we observe and what we infer). We observe with the corporeal eye, we infer with the eye of reason, and with this eye of reason we can penetrate into hidden recesses where the corporeal eye will not reach. The earlier physicians, of course, had a naive idea of perception. They did not use the word in the sense of modern psychology. Instead they spoke of experience, which they contrasted with reason. And by experience they meant, in Boerhaave's words, something "observable by the aid of the senses. Our mind adds nothing to the phenomenon beyond its bare perception."[11]

In the earlier formulations we saw that the disease, as the cause, produced the symptoms, as effect. Can we retrace the steps and from the observation of symptoms infer their cause— the disease? If we do so, then the symptoms—the manifestations—are the signs of the disease. When we observe the phenomena *and* interpret them, then the phenomena become signs. Unless we interpret them, the symptoms remain symptoms.

The older authors identified four types of signs, depending on the inferences to which they gave rise. A prognostic sign indicates not the name of the disease but the clinical outcome of a given bodily state. The most famous example of a prognostic sign is the "Hippocratic facies," whereby Hippocrates described impending death: ". . . the nose sharp, the eyes sunken, the temples fallen in, the ears cold . . . , the colour of the face pale or dusky . . . if there is no improvement, . . . this sign portends death."[12] These various features which Hippocrates described were the result of the disease. Hippocrates, however, used these observations to infer not the name of the disease but rather its outcome. Indeed, his writings on prognosis are among his most famous and influential works. He indicated to physicians which signs meant a favorable outcome and which ones an unfavorable one. The prognostic signs were pointing to the future.

Other signs can point to the past, to some disease or condition that existed formerly and has left its present traces. From observation of these present phenomena we can infer the nature of the disease that was responsible. We see a man walking with a paralyzed arm and a characteristic gait, and we say, "This man had a stroke." We see a picture on an old Egyptian stele dating back to 1500 B.C. depicting a man with one shrivelled leg, and we have no hesitation in saying that this man had suffered an attack of poliomyelitis, from which he recovered. This type of sign the older physicians called anamnestic.

Most common, and most important, were the signs called "diagnostic," referring to the disease from which the patient is currently suffering. These are the signs that lead the physician to make a diagnosis—and in many instances the layman can also make a diagnosis. The grandmother who had herself brought up a large family may be able to diagnose the measles in her grandchild before the doctor arrives. Of course, she may be wrong, but, then, doctors too are often wrong.

Diagnostic signs lead to the recognition and identification of a disease. The fourth type of sign, called pathognomonic, is any phenomenon whose presence meant, beyond any reasonable doubt, that a particular disease was present. It is, so to speak, a marked intensification of a diagnostic sign.

In summary of the older views, we see that a symptom is a phenomenon, caused by an illness and observable directly in experience. We may speak of it as a *manifestation* of illness. When the observer reflects on that phenomenon and uses it as a base for further inferences, then that symptom is transformed into a sign. As a sign it points beyond itself—perhaps to the present illness, or to the past or to the future. That to which a sign points is part of its meaning, which may be rich and complex, or scanty, or any gradation in between.

In medicine, then, a sign is thus a phenomenon from which we may get a message, a message that tells us something about the patient or the disease. A phenomenon or observation that does not convey a message is not a sign. The distinction between signs and symptom rests on the meaning, and this is not perceived but inferred.

## III

What we now call physical diagnosis had its essential beginning in the early 19th century with the introduction of percussion and auscultation. To be sure, Auenbrugger had developed percussion as a diagnostic tool in the 18th century, but it was not popularized until 1808, when Corvisart translated the original work into French. Then, in 1816 Laennec invented the first crude stethoscope, which he later refined, and first published his findings in 1819. With these procedures of percussion and auscultation, new techniques entered medical practice and profoundly altered traditional ideas. The new technology allowed the distinction of subjective and objective and added a new dimension to the relations of physicians to patients.

In an earlier and simpler era the important data for making a diagnosis came in part from the history given by the patient and in part from surface observations. Prior to the 19th century the physician paid considerable attention to what the patient himself noticed, for in general there was not a great deal of difference between what the patient perceived and what the doctor perceived. The great difference between the physician and the patient lay in interpretation. The physician knew what the findings *meant* and the layman did not. Because of his background knowledge the various observations could disclose a meaning hidden from the layman. We might compare the observations to a sentence written in a language the patient did not understand. But for the man who knew the language the words did spell out a meaning.

Before the advent of technological advances, any notion of subjective, as contrasted with objective, was quite pointless. The important contrast lay in the degree of understanding to which the observations might give rise. The physician had understanding, the patient did not. The physician would draw inferences from what he observed, the patient could not. Physician and patient could both note a swelling or a discoloration or a deformity but would differ in their ability to interpret, or to assign significance.

The introduction of percussion and auscultation changed all

that, for these techniques *affected the capacity to observe*. The patient did not have a stethoscope and did not know how to thump a chest. The physician did. A sound is a datum of observation just as much as the visual perception of swelling or discoloration. But, whereas both patient and physician could see a swelling, a sound did not enter consciousness unbidden. Something had to be done to the patient to elicit a sound. Only a physician could do the necessary manipulation to elicit the phenomena.

Of course, even if the patient did hear the sound, he would not know what it meant. The sound had to be interpreted; it was raw material for inference. The physician thus had a double advantage over the layman. Only the physician could elicit the data, and only he could interpret them. Thus, through new technical advances, a class of phenomena became peculiarly associated with the activity of the physician. Some new name might seem desirable for data accessible to the physicians but not to the patient, some name that would distinguish these observations from others accessible to the patient as well. The term "signs" seemed appropriate for the former class, "symptoms" for the latter.

## IV

In the years following the invention of the stethoscope, the medical profession had to learn how to use the instrument, distinguish the various sounds and grasp their significance. In examination of the lungs, for example, one type of sound might mean moisture in the air sacs; a different one might indicate consolidation; a still different one, that a cavity was present. Many times the differences between sounds might be quite slight and observers might not agree on the meaning conveyed.

The new technology appealed chiefly to the younger physicians, while many of the older generation showed considerable resistance. The actual manipulations were not difficult, but finding out what the sounds really meant required learning a whole new language, a task difficult for middle-aged physicians. The steps by which auscultation finally became fully accepted is an interesting chapter in medical, social, and cultural history.[13] Eventually instruction in auscultation was incorporated in the medical school curriculum, and the procedure became a standard method of examination. The students were taught the new language, intelligible only to the initiated. Initiation began in medical school.

The stethoscope allows inferential knowledge of what is happening in the lungs during life. A far more powerful tool than the stethoscope is the x-ray, developed at the turn of the 20th century. This mode of examination, one of the great triumphs of modern science, provides a series of shadows whose density corresponds quite accurately to the varied densities of the bodily tissues. The radiologist does not see the lungs or other parts of the body with his corporeal eye. He sees shadows that he interprets through a process of inference.

I would emphasize the similarities between auscultation and radiological examination. Both provide indirect knowledge reached by interpretation. In either modality the raw data, if presented to the untrained layman—the sounds in the one case, the shadows in the other—would not convey much of any meaning, would not give rise to inference, and would not constitute signs.

The microscope is another tool for amassing indirect knowledge. Bits of tissue, when sectioned and stained, can convey a great deal of information to the pathologist, but none at all to the untrained person who happens to look into the microscope. A microscopic slide is entirely comparable to the x-ray film. The trained physician who studies the patterns, shades, and colors under the microscope is making indirect observations of a part of the body. The various colors and shadings, lines and dots, do not exist as such in the body, but they have a *correspondence* to what does exist, a correspondence that can be inferred and given meaning by suitable interpretation. The patterns that the physician sees in the colored transparencies allow him to make interpretations, so that he finds diagnostic, prognostic, and anamnestic signs in the material he examines.

Auscultation, radiology, and microscopy, even though they

differ markedly in their techniques, all give indirect information about the structure of the body. In the 19th and 20th centuries science and technology also produced complicated apparatus that permitted direct visual observation of hidden parts of
the body. The ophthalmoscope, which allows the observer to
examine directly the interior of the eye, will serve as prototype
of numerous other "-scopes" that give direct visual access to
concealed areas: larynx, bladder, rectum, stomach, and so on.

The physician who wanted to use such instruments had to
have special training, in part to acquire the manipulative techniques but, even more important, to distinguish the normal
from the abnormal and to learn the inferences to which the
observations might lead. He had to identify, discriminate, and
interpret the visual impressions that the instruments furnished.

So far I have distinguished the direct from the indirect methods of perceiving changes in the body. Direct methods would
include visual observation of the surface of the body (as in the
examination by a dermatologist), or the interior of the body (as
by an ophthalmologist or gastroscopist). Indirect observation involves instruments such as the x-ray or the microscope, whereby
the observer studies not the body itself but the symbolic representation of the bodily parts, whether through sounds, shadows,
or chemically treated snippets.

Yet the different methods, direct as well as indirect, have
certain features in common: sensory presentations that require
interpretation. The dermatologist sees changes in color, contour,
texture, and general appearance of the skin; the ophthalmologist
studies analogous changes in the eye; the auscultator notes
changes in the breath sounds transmitted through the chest wall;
the radiologist sees congeries of shadows; the pathologist notes
patterns and details of colored masses. The difficulty lies not in
seeing or hearing, but in understanding, i.e., in drawing conclusions from what is seen or heard.

So far the data requiring interpretation have been drawn from
the structural aspects of the body. Other information derives
from the study of function.

Perhaps the simplest mode of examining a bodily function is

feeling the pulse. The observer can count the rate and attend to the various qualities. Common descriptive terms might be: strong, full, bounding, forceful, weak, thready, feeble, irregular, intermittent, and so on. Older physicians, especially in the Orient, might spend a long time feeling various pulses, whose properties gradually acquired a great deal of meaning. The rate and qualities of the pulse became signs from which the older physicians would draw conclusions, which in turn might lead to surprisingly accurate diagnoses.

In the 19th century many new ways of studying the heart gradually developed. Most common today is the electrocardiogram (EKG), wherein the electrical activity of the heart is transformed into linear records. To the untrained person the apparatus produces only meaningless squiggles, yet the tracings are a symbolic representation—a correspondence—relating functional activity with a series of marks. Obviously, special training is necessary to interpret the various jagged lines and to invest them with meaning.

I have repeatedly compared the interpretation of medical data with translating a foreign language. We can appreciate the aptness of the parallel if we contrast a layman looking at an x-ray film with the same layman seeing an EKG tracing. An x-ray film examined by a layman would be comparable to a French text seen by a person who does not know French. He might, however, grasp a few words here and there through their similarity to English. In comparable fashion, the technical "language" of the x-ray may, on occasion, have enough relation to everyday experience to permit some plausible guesses. Thus, almost any layman would correctly identify an x-ray showing a broken long bone with marked displacement. However, to the untutored layman the EKG tracing (or an electroencephalogram) would be comparable to a text in Chinese. They would both elicit the same bewilderment.

Modern chemistry can provide an enormous amount of information regarding bodily functions. The data that it provides are highly abstract, consisting only of a number—a quantitative value, referring ordinarily to relative volume or weight, or else

to a purely arbitrary standard. Anyone, even an untrained layman, can read a number, but that is of little importance. We
want to know what the number *means*. Can we invest it with
*significance*, i.e., let it serve as a sign? But a sign of what?

If a patient has a blood sugar of, say, 160 milligrams per
hundred cubic centimeters of blood, he wants to know what that
means. Is it a sign of diabetes? The answer would necessarily
be, "That all depends." A vast number of factors bear on the
interpretation of a number and any conclusion that fails to take
them into account runs great risk of error. With chemical data
that reflect the functional state of the body, evaluation and interpretation may be more difficult, more uncertain, than with data
regarding structure.


### V

Originally, as we have seen, a symptom meant a manifestation
of disease, a change in the body brought about by the disease.
The disease was, so to speak, the cause, the symptom the effect.
And, just as the study of an effect may enable us to infer the
cause, so the study of symptoms could lead us back to the disease
itself. When the symptoms thus give rise to inference, they become signs. But if no conclusion is drawn, the symptom remains
a symptom, at best only a potential sign.

Beginning in the early 19th century, improved technology
enabled physicians to discover new and unsuspected manifestations of disease—disturbances in both structure and function, of
a complexity undreamed of in an earlier era. This wealth of new
observations had profound effects. I would merely point to the
new categories that physicians created to accommodate the data:
physical signs, radiological signs, signs from chemistry, clinical
pathology, bacteriology and anatomical pathology. The original
distinction of signs and symptoms, clear enough to the early
physicians, became obscured by the mass of data from special
examinations and tests.

It is illuminating, in this connection, to note the comments
written in 1864 by the Philadelphia physician J. M. da Costa.
He entitled his book, *Medical Diagnosis With Special Reference*

*to Practical Medicine*, with the subtitle, "Guide to the Knowledge and Discrimination of Diseases." He wrote at a time when substantial advances had already been made in our knowledge of disease, and when much special technology was already available to the physician; yet, when he wrote, medical science was barely on the threshold of the progress still to come. If the reader will refer to Chapter 2 above, on Consumption, he will appreciate the progress that had already been made by 1864, and also the progress that science was yet to make in the subsequent years. Da Costa's remarks represent a half-way house, intermediate between simplistic 18th-century medicine and the complexity of the late 20th century.

"The detection of disease," he said, "is the product of the close observation of symptoms, and of correct deduction from these symptoms. . . . Now, to recognize the manifestations of disease, [regardless] *whether they are or are not readily perceptible*, we have to employ our eyes and ears, our sense of touch and smell. Formerly we could go no further than these senses unassisted would carry us. But science has lent its aid, and furnished means by the help of which we can detect clearly what before we could not detect at all. . . . The microscope gives at a glance insight into matters far beyond anything the naked eye discloses. And chemistry, with its marvellous teachings, is rendering our knowledge of many morbid states admirable and amazingly complete. . . ." He went on: "When, by means of the aided or unaided senses, the symptoms of the malady have been discovered, the next step toward a diagnosis is a proper appreciation of their significance and of their relation toward each other. Knowledge, and, above all, the exercise of the reasoning faculties, are now indispensable. . . ."[14]

Da Costa's language emphasizes a time-honored view: that the malady manifests itself through symptoms. Certain of these manifestations the patient himself recognizes; others the physician can identify by his unaided senses; still others he can identify by the use of technical aids, such as the stethoscope. New technology made available new procedures that could give information about the cellular and chemical composition of the blood, the urine, and other fluids and dejecta. More recent apparatus has extended the range of observation into areas of fantastic subtlety.

The results of such examinations could be normal or abnormal (or doubtful). The abnormal findings, as da Costa indicated, would be evidence of disease. The proper terminology for such evidence would be symptoms. The symptoms would thus include the results from whatever modality supplied the data—microscopy, chemistry, the senses, whether unaided or aided. His view harmonizes with the first definition of "symptom" found in the 1900 edition of Dorland's *American Illustrated Dictionary*: "any evidence of disease or of a patient's condition." The words *any evidence* are crucial.[15]

The distinction became more intense as technology became more and more important. Perhaps to the physician intoxicated with the glories of "scientific" medicine the term "symptom" appeared old-fashioned and some further term seemed desirable to identify the sophisticated data of modern technology. Nevertheless, as da Costa implied, *symptoms should include abnormal laboratory data, as manifestations of disease*, as well as the patient's subjective complaints and the physician's observations.

The belief that a symptom is a subjective report of the patient, while a sign is something that the physician elicits, is a 20th-century product that contravenes the usage of two thousand years of medicine. In practice, now as always, the physician makes his judgments from the information that he gathers. The modern usage of signs and symptoms emphasizes merely the source of the information, which is not really too important. Far more important is the use that the information serves. If the data, however derived, lead to some inferences and go beyond themselves, those data are signs. If, however, the data remain as mere observations without interpretation, they are symptoms, regardless of their source. Symptoms become signs when they lead to an interpretation. The distinction between information and inference underlies all medical thinking and should be preserved. The modern riot of technology has given rise to linguistic usage that obscures clear thinking.

## CHAPTER 4

# Diagnosis

*Diagnosis is central to the practice of medicine*, for it identifies the disease from which the patient suffers. Much of medical education centers around the problem: how do you learn to make a diagnosis? One recent text gave this advice: the student should "begin, as in all scientific research, by marshalling all the facts, then proceeding with an unprejudiced analysis of facts, and end with a logical conclusion."[1]

I would point out the similarity of this excellent advice to that which da Costa offered more than a century before (see p. 88). Da Costa indicated the following steps: discover the "symptoms" (i.e., the "facts"), then "appreciate" their significance (i.e., regard them as *signs* that point somewhere). For this purpose the student must use his "reasoning faculties." These steps are identical in essence, if not in wording, with the present-day recommendations.

Many authors describe ways of making a diagnosis, but only a few discuss the basic concepts, what diagnosis *is*, and how it relates to other essential terms in medicine.[2] Presentation of their views would involve extensive argument, which I wish to avoid. Hence I will simply present my own views without analyzing the recent literature.

Diagnosis identifies the disease from which the patient suffers. The process has its roots in classification, a complex term that I will analyze in greater detail in the next chapter. Suffice now to indicate its essential nature: establishing a series of classes. These serve as pigeonholes or compartments, each with its own distinguishing properties. We have, so to speak, a series of empty spaces, each with a label, and we also have an indiscriminate mass of entities that we may want to put into those

spaces. Someone must decide whether any given object belongs
in any given space. Diagnosis consists in deciding which object
goes into which niche of the framework. It is a process of fitting
individuals into appropriate containers—a practical activity that
requires judgment.

Various dictionaries and various individual writers give other
definitions. There are three main variants: diagnosis distinguishes one disease from another, or it identifies the disease, or
it determines the nature of the disease. The subtle differences
between these views all ignore one crucial point—that, while
diagnosis now has a chiefly medical context, in its essence it is
not a medical term at all but has a vastly broader meaning.
Unless we grasp this broader sense we cannot appreciate the
medical sense.

From its derivation diagnosis means to distinguish. This involves discrimination. Whenever I say that *this* (regardless of
what *this* might be) is an example of *that* (regardless of what
*that* might be), I am making a diagnosis. If I say "This is a
rose," I am making a diagnosis just as surely as when I say,
"This is cancer of the breast."

In diagnosis we find three essential features. First, there must
exist a series of classes or categories, among which the choice
rests. In the realm of flowers we have roses and dahlias and
peonies, and thousands of others. When I say, "This is a rose,"
I am at the same time saying that it is not a dahlia or a peony.
Similarly, in a medical diagnosis, when I say "This is cancer of
the breast," I am at the same time saying that it is not diabetes
or Parkinson's disease, or any of the other conditions we find in
the medical textbooks.

The first requirement, then, for a diagnosis is an available
series of classes, as the framework within which the choice is to
be made. The second requirement is the particular object,
whether it is a flower or a human patient, that is going to be
placed in one or another of the categories. And, third, before
we make the actual assignment to a class, we have the reflection
and discrimination, that makes us say, "*This* object belongs in
*that* category and not in any other." The decision may require

careful study and long reflection, or it may occur immediately, almost reflexly.

## The Framework

In medicine there is a great temptation to take for granted some "standard" framework of diseases, such as we might find in the latest edition of a textbook of medicine. However, the process we call diagnosis is the same, whether we have two categories or many thousands. We must have a least two, for otherwise there can be no choice, but there is no upper limit. In diagnostic decisions the number of relevant classes among which the choice must rest will depend on context and circumstances. Let me give some examples.

I knew a highly educated professional man who had great faith in modern medicine. When he was ill he did not ask his physician about the diagnosis in the conventional sense. He wanted his physician to answer only one question: "Do I have something to worry about?" In this instance the diagnostic framework had only two niches—diseases with something to worry about, and those with nothing to worry about. In this context the physician had to decide into which of these two categories his patient fitted. The decision is a diagnostic process just as truly as if the doctor, after much travail, had decided, "You are suffering from gnathostomiasis."

An act of diagnosis limited to three categories we find in certain emergency situations, whether in warfare or in civilian disasters. In the process known as triage someone must make a decision that involves not the name of the injury but rather the priority for treatment. There are only three classes: the patients for whom there is no hope of recovery, those who should get immediate treatment, and those who can wait. Does this patient have a mortal injury? Should that patient have priority over someone else? Whoever makes the decision is making a diagnosis—a discrimination according to particular criteria.

In ancient Egypt the surgeons also practiced triage, with a threefold division of diseases: those they would treat, those they would "contend with," and those ailments "not to be treated."

These three classes had the following criteria: conditions the surgeons felt confident of curing, those they hoped to cure but about which they had reservations, and those they regarded as hopeless.

There is historical warrant for a framework of only four classes. In the 18th century the German physician J. G. Zimmermann described a colleague who had such a division. "I knew a certain Esculapius," he said, "who has 50 or 60 patients every morning in his anti-chamber. He just listens a moment to the complaints of each, and then arranges them in four divisions. To the first, he prescribes blood-letting; to the second, a purge; to the third, a clyster; and to the fourth, change of air."[3] The diagnostic categories are characterized not by the name of the disease but by the treatment handed out. This type of medical practice is by no means unknown today, although blood-letting, purging, and clysters have perhaps given way to antibiotics, steroids, and tranquillizers.

### The Object Diagnosed

As our second point we may properly ask: "What is it that we are diagnosing?" Let us assume that a clinician, after examining a patient, makes a diagnosis of myocardial infarction. While the medical study points to the heart as the locus of the acute illness, it is the patient who is being subjected to study. It is the patient who suffers from cardiac infarction.

We may contrast this with the actions of the pathologist who receives a biopsy specimen taken from a patient suspected of having a cancer of the breast. The pathologist examines the specimen grossly and microscopically and then makes his diagnosis: fibrocystic disease of the breast. Clearly, in this case the pathologist is studying the specimen, not the patient.

A comparable example: a patient scheduled for surgery may need a transfusion. The technician brings down a sample of blood for typing. The sample is characterized as Group A, Rh negative (ignoring all other specifications). The pathologist cannot say that the patient is Group A, Rh negative. All he can say is that the sample was so characterized. Rarely a sample of blood is mislabelled, and gets attributed to the wrong person. We must keep clearly in mind just what entity is being fitted into the appropriate niche in the diagnostic framework.

## The Process of Decision

The third aspect is the act of commitment, the ultimate decision, that the object does in fact fit into this or that category. Jevons, in 1892, gave an idealized account of the process: "Diagnosis consists in comparing the qualities of a certain object with the definitions of a series of classes; the absence in the object of any one quality stated in the definition excludes it from the class thus defined; whereas, if we find every point of a definition exactly fulfilled in the specimen, we may at once assign it to the class in question." The diagnosis, of course, does not consist merely in a comparison but rather in the decision made after the comparison has taken place.[4]

Jevons' concept is well illustrated by the example already mentioned: identifying an unfamiliar flower. To accomplish this, we ordinarily rely on some authority, usually a book that will describe the different flowers of the region. Then we must determine whether the flower in hand matches some description in the book. Finding an answer will depend on two variables: the knowledge and skill of the questioner and the type of book. The book, whatever it is, will provide a series of classes, preferably in some sort of hierarchical order, and for each class will give the identifying marks, whether verbal or pictorial or both. Let us examine two contrasting examples.

There are admirable guides that assume no technical knowledge of botany. One excellent volume has only three hierarchical steps. The first division is by color—white, yellow, blue, and so on. Under each of these primary groupings there are subsidiary classes that offer various configurations of flowers or leaves, such as "umbrella-like cluster, finely cut leaves"; or "showy spikes and pannicles"; or "lipped, lobed, tubular flowers"; or "sunflower-like plants with large leaves." For each of these groupings (which provide rough subdivisions) there is a third and final hierarchical step, namely, half a dozen or so individual examples, with illustrations and brief verbal description.[5]

This deservedly popular book classifies plants not by family, genus, and species, but by color and configuration of the flowers. It enables those with no knowledge of botany to find the *names* of a great many wildflowers, and then, once the name is known, additional knowledge can readily be acquired. Everyone who uses this book is engaged in the process of diagnosis as Jevons describes it. The diagnostician compares the qualities in his flower with those enumerated in the book. If he finds that the flower fits, he can "at once assign it to the class in question." And then he knows the name of the flower and he has achieved his diagnosis.

The skilled botanist who finds an unfamiliar flower that he wants to identify also engages in a process of diagnosis. He too must answer the question as to whether the flower matches a description in a book, but he relies on a very different book whose arrangement accords with the best botanical principles and is couched in a technical vocabulary.

To discriminate among many possibilities, the botanist may use a key. This is an aspect of so-called branching logic that offers a sequence of choices, each narrowing the field and leading to a further choice, in a continuous branching arrangement. The presence or absence of some particular property gradually eliminates various possibilities and brings the searcher closer and closer to the answer he is seeking.

A botanical key is comparable to a road that branches repeatedly but has markers at each division. If the signposts are accurate and clear and if the traveler reads them correctly, he will reach his destination. However, quite possibly the directions are not entirely accurate, or perhaps the traveler does not read them properly. Then he will lose his way. With a well-constructed key the botanist will soon eliminate all but a few classes. Then, as Jevons indicated, he notes the criteria described in the text and compares them with the corresponding features in the flower. Finally comes the definitive judgment: "This is an example of that class." This final commitment is the act of diagnosis.

In the practice of medicine, branching logic and the use of keys are finding more and more application, especially in the realm of computer diagnosis and algorithms. These relatively new techniques permit physicians to consider various possibilities systematically and to evaluate them through the presence or absence of discrete criteria. I will not enter the controversy as to whether the computer or algorithms can substitute for intuitive judgment. In the 17th century Francis Bacon devised a method of noting similarities and differences, with a systematic comparison. His method, he thought, "goes far to level men's wits, and leaves but little to individual excellence; because it performs everything by the surest rules and demonstrations."[6] However, events did not work out as Bacon had expected. Perhaps algorithms will not fulfill expectations either.

In the 18th century Boerhaave recognized explicitly the need for due reflection on the findings. When he wrote, the logic of diagnosis had not yet received much attention and he used a different vocabulary than we would today. The concepts, however, are comparable. He described the way an 18th-century physician should approach the process of decision-making:

"At first visiting the patient, unless the physician is perfectly clear in the case, he ought to speak in general terms, not capable of being taken hold of, and order some innocent medicine." (That is, he should not commit himself in any way when he is not sure.) The physician should, however, make "a memorandum at the same time of all the symptoms upon a piece of paper, that he may at home more leisurely weigh them in his mind." (That is, he should analyze the symptoms—i.e., manifestations—in unhurried fashion and, as Harvey and Bordley recommended two and a half centuries later, "end with a logical conclusion.") For Boerhaave this meant that he should "determine with himself which is the part affected; in what stage the disease is advanced; what may be thence feared; upon what part the disorder may be translated, etc. Thus, he will always be able to understand the disease, having first rightly considered all the circumstances; but if this method be neglected he will always be liable to error and mistake."[7]

This can readily be transformed into thoroughly modern terms. If the physician is not immediately sure of the diagnosis, he should not commit himself and should temporize until he has had a chance to reflect and discriminate. *The modern physician does exactly this*, but, instead of meditating at home as did Boerhaave, he puts the patient in the hospital, orders laboratory work, and asks for consultations.

## Rapid Diagnosis

In ordinary medical practice, most cases are not great puzzles. The proper diagnosis may be almost immediately apparent with only a modest degree of reflection, and the conscientious physician will then use various procedures as merely confirmatory. Some diagnoses are made with assurance immediately on inspection. The dermatologist takes one look at a young patient with acne and at once makes the presumptive identification; the internist notes a characteristic gait and posture and instantly says that the patient had a "stroke." Similarly, the pathologist examining a series of slides takes one glance at a florid carcinoma of the breast and at once gives the diagnosis. Thus, in certain instances the physician will achieve an immediate diagnosis that is a non-reflective identification. How does this non-reflective diagnosis relate to the more labored process that we have considered?

Immediate recognition is, in part, a function of familiarity, as we find in almost any modality. If, on an autumn day, we walk on a tree-lined street, we will see abundant fallen leaves. Most of us have no hesitation in picking up, say, a maple leaf, and identifying it. Of all the varied properties that characterize the genus *acer*, the shape of the leaves is quite characteristic, and the leaves of the common species are not likely to get confused with the leaves of other genera. If we make the effort, we can learn to identify a wide range of trees simply by examining their leaves. Behind this experience there lurk some important presuppositions, significant for medicine and the diagnostic process.

In identifying trees by their leaves we attend to a limited pattern—the configuration of the leaf—and we know that this is merely a part, an intrinsic and organic part, of a larger pattern, namely, the properties of the tree as a whole. We know that the single part—the leaf—serves as an *index* of the whole. For purposes of identification, recognizing the part is the equivalent of recognizing the whole.

The equivalence of the part for the whole is a concept thoroughly familiar in ordinary language, in the figure of speech known as "metonymy." Thus, we may speak of the "tube" when we refer to the television receiver; or to "strings" for a group of instruments in an orchestra; or to "hands" for workers on the farm or in the factory.

Metonymy, however, has an arbitrary quality dependent on context. "Strings" mean one thing in reference to an orchestra, something quite different in relation to political influence. In a florist's shop or plant nursery, "flats" mean something quite different than what they mean in a shoestore. On the other hand, when we say that a particular type of leaf represents a particular type of tree, there is nothing arbitrary involved, and no dependence on artificial context. The "belonging" of a part to the whole is a "natural" phenomenon, where organic connections are quite distinct from the arbitrary connections that we find in language. This distinction between "natural" and "artificial" has great historical and theoretical importance in both biology and medicine, and will be further discussed in the next chapter.

If we return now to the immediate or non-reflective diagnosis, we see that it rests on a concealed premise: that the features taken in at a glance comprise an intrinsic part of an organic pattern; further, that the observed part is connected with only one whole, without ambiguity or confusion. The leaf of the silver maple, for example, has an unambiguous relation to the silver maple tree, and not with the Norway maple or the pin oak.

In reference to medicine, if a dermatologist takes one look at an adolescent and diagnoses acne, the manifestations noted at a glance would have a relationship comparable to the relation of the leaf to the silver maple tree. Just as the leaf is part of the total pattern of the tree, so the age of the patient and the type and distribution of the lesions are part of the total pattern we call acne.

*The Pathognomonic Sign*

At this point we should note briefly the concept of the pathognomonic sign mentioned previously, and its connection with the
diagnostic pattern and the rapid diagnosis. In Boerhaave's writings, which we will take as an example, diseases were considered
distinct entities. Every disease was different from every other
and could be distinguished by its signs (*per sua signa dignosci
potest*). The pathognomonic sign is that which is "characteristic
(*proprium*) of the disease, inseparable from it, as arising from its
nature." Boerhaave went on to explain that a pathognomonic
sign is characteristic of one disease and does not fit any other.
When this sign is known, the disease cannot be confused with
any other.[8]

Boerhaave wished that such signs were available for every
disease, but, unfortunately, he went on, in all of medicine we
have such signs in only three or four diseases. For example, he
said, in a bladder stone the pathognomonic sign is touching it
with a catheter. For the modern reader this example will bear
some elaboration. A patient who had a bladder stone would show
various manifestations. Thus, he could have difficulty in uri-
nation and varying amounts of pain, symptoms (manifestations)
that have the technical name "dysuria." He also might have
some blood or pus in the urine, the results of inflammation that
the stone had set up. These features constitute signs that point
to the bladder as the locus of the disease. But the bladder can be
the site of many different diseases, and these symptoms are in
no way specific. They could arise not only from stone but from
such conditions as prostatic enlargement with infection and inflammation, or tumor, or drugs (e.g., cantharides, often used
as an aphrodisiac but often inducing inflammation of the bladder). How could the physician tell *which* disease existed in the
bladder? In modern terminology he was facing a problem of
differential diagnosis—determining which of several possibilities actually existed.

The 18th-century physician could not inspect the inside of the
bladder through a cystoscope. In the case of bladder stone, however, he did have a means of discrimination. He could pass a
catheter into the bladder. If this catheter (made of metal or

wood, not of soft rubber) struck the stone, there would result a characteristic sense of resistance that the experienced physician would easily recognize. This special sensation would not appear with any of the other possible diseases that might produce the symptoms. Hence, in the face of multiple non-specific symptoms, the passing of a catheter permitted a sharp discrimination. A positive finding in this respect meant, unequivocally, that the patient had stone in the bladder. No other disease would give this finding, which thus became a pathognomonic sign.

Symptoms become signs when they permit inference. Ordinarily, one single symptom by itself—such as pain or swelling, or discoloration, or bloody discharge—would not permit any specific inference, but when symptoms occur in clusters and form a pattern, then the aggregate might point to a particular disease. The pathognomonic sign, however, does not need any other manifestation to lead the physician to the correct diagnosis. It constitutes a one-to-one relationship—the sign and the disease are uniquely related. The pathognomonic sign was the "clincher," the datum that established the diagnosis unequivocally.

### Changes in Diagnostic Categories

In medical history the total number of diagnostic categories propounded at one or another time is truly staggering. Of the various terms some have disappeared entirely; others have persisted but with greater or less change in meaning. New terms might or might not gain general acceptance. Categories do not remain static but get progressively modified as new experience and new theories exert their influence. We can advantageously study some of these changes. I will limit myself to a few aspects of cancer, especially cancer of the breast.

This tumor, in its full-blown state, has been well recognized since antiquity. The properties of a hard swelling, destructive invasion, ulceration, pain, and fatal outcome were quite characteristic. By the 18th century advanced cancer was quite clearly defined, but the early stages were not readily identified.

In addition to cancer, physicians identified a benign tumor of the breast, called "scirrhus," that might transform into the malignant state. According to Boerhaave and his pupil van Swieten, a scirrhus was a painless hard swelling that arose in glandular tissue, from blockage of secretions, so that the secreted substances became confined in the glandular follicles and ducts and then hardened. The female breast was a favorite site, but comparable lesions could occur in any glandular organ such as the lips, uterus, pancreas, and the like.

Van Swieten declared, "A scirrhus is of itself inoffensive, but it frequently becomes malignant or cancerous." By way of explanation he declared, "The concreted humours . . . which have hitherto lain in a mild unactive state in their containing obstructed vessels or receptacles, begin to corrupt or putrefy, and acquire a greater acrimony, by which they may be capable of irritating or corroding the parts in which they are contained." If the tumor becomes painful, starts to erode and ulcerate, these are signs of malignant change. "The concreted substances of the scirrhus itself may at length become spontaneously acrid," and then it can corrode. We must remember, of course, that the author had no knowledge of cell theory.[9]

In 1759 Jean Astruc (1684-1766) gave a somewhat more detailed and analytical description. He indicated five characteristic signs of a scirrhus: it is hard and resistant; it is indolent; it does not alter the normal color of the site; there is no accompanying heat; and it is formed by a gradual slow congestion. He distinguished six different kinds or "species." The "perfect" scirrhus showed all the features of the definition: it was hard and resistant, indolent, without special heat or change of color. Other species might be less resistant or show twinges of pain and a changing configuration, or have some degree of inflammatory change or lack circumscription.

In a vague way Astruc pointed to many kinds of swellings that differed one from the other. In retrospect, we see that he was trying to distinguish inflammatory swellings from neoplasms, and, among neoplasms, the benign from the malignant. These concepts, however, had not yet been articulated, and he could not furnish any sound basis for classification. He had no sharp criteria. In the 18th century the scirrhus was a vaguely conceptualized group of tumors. Many cases would go on to obvious cancer but many would not, and there was no good way to differentiate those which did from those which did not. The diagnostic category was not precise.[10]

The concept of scirrhus included a wide range of lesions having in common a more or less painless growth and a hard consistency. Today we know that these might include such widely diverse lesions as fibromas, leiomyomas, cysts, fibroadenomas, some hyperplastic changes, instances of chronic inflammation, and, of course, some true carcinomas at an early stage. Each of these would have its own course and prognosis. Astruc was quite aware that the swellings in the category scirrhus did not form a homogeneous class, but he could not provide any adequate means of discrimination.

Advances in the non-clinical sciences gradually rendered obsolete the older concept of scirrhus. Bichat, at the turn of the 19th century, had focused attention on the individual tissues, for the study of which microscopy and cell theory brought about revolutionary advances. With a knowledge of microscopic anatomy pathologists would distinguish different kinds of tumors, identify their origins, and correlate their appearance and behavior with certain types of cells. Precise new observational data could help to distinguish benign from malignant. In all this new movement, Rudolph Virchow was a prominent leader.

By the last quarter of the 19th century the main lines of progress were well established. Inflammation was clearly demarcated from neoplasms, and benign tumors were, in a general fashion, separated into different kinds, corresponding to the tissues or origin. By 1889 Delafield and Prudden had distinguished many different benign tumors of the breast—cysts, fibromas, intracanalicular fibromas, myxomas, chondromas, adenomas.[11]

In the 18th century these would have all been lumped together as scirrhus of the breast, for they were all hard and virtually painless. But with the recognition of cell-specific tumors the category scirrhus no longer served a useful function. It no longer had any value as an organizing principle for interpreting experience.

By the last quarter of the 19th century considerable progress had also been made in analyzing definite cancer of the breast. Delafield and Prudden separated three main types. The criteria were simple. In the first group, called medullary cancer, the tumor consisted principally of epithelial cells and the consistency was therefore relatively soft. In another type the cells were relatively sparse and the connective tissue stroma predominated. This tumor, hard and dense, was called a scirrhous cancer. An intermediate group, where cells and stroma were developed about equally, was designated carcinoma simplex. (The authors also identified a rare type that need not concern us, a "colloid" carcinoma that contained extensive mucin.) The nomenclature, when translated into simple English, meant that the cancers were soft or hard or intermediate—no profound advance on Astruc.

## Usefulness of Diagnostic Categories

In the most general terms diagnosis consists of fitting an individual specimen into one or another category or class. These classes represent the framework within which the diagnostician operates. The actual process of diagnosis lies in assigning an individual to an appropriate category. And the word "appropriate" refers to the purpose for which the diagnosis is carried out. In medicine we ordinarily associate diagnosis with the physician in practice, who treats sick people. Here the specimen is the individual patient and the classes represent different diseases. The clinician tries to place the patient in the proper category so that he can institute therapy. In botany, on the other hand, the specimen would be an individual flower or plant and the framework would be the whole taxonomic arrangement in all its subdivisions.

The medical historian must take into account the profound changes among diagnostic categories, as we have already noted in reference to cancer and scirrhus. This process of change becomes somewhat easier to interpret when we appreciate the way that specialization has increased. Specialists create their own particular frameworks and make them ever more detailed and precise. Increased precision in one branch may influence the classification in some other branch. Thus, increased knowledge of microscopic appearances of tumors can influence the diagnostic and therapeutic choice that the surgeon makes. However, the surgeon or internist will draw on the diagnostic categories of various specialists only when usefulness has been proved. For the clinician, "use" refers to the value in promoting cure. In research, however, "use" might mean the value in promoting understanding.

Specialty groups will elaborate their own arrangement of classes according to their particular needs. We must appreciate, however, the complex interactions affecting diagnostic categories. Of the different variables one would be the intrinsic subject matter of the specialty; another, the degree of precision useful in that specialty; another, the cross-influence exerted by other groups. There is no sharp line of division, but all flow one into the others as the occasion requires. Thus, in one context a simple distinction between benign and malignant may be quite adequate and satisfactory. If, for example, an x-ray disclosed a tumor of the lung, the patient would naturally fear a malignancy. If the tumor on removal proved to be benign, the surgeon and the patient might be entirely satisfied with that diagnostic category, however lacking in detail. The pathologist might feel quite differently. If the tumor were a relatively unusual lesion, such as, say, a hamartoma, the pathologist would fall back on a complex diagnostic framework, important to him although not to the surgeon.

Diagnosis is, in a sense, the reverse of classification and intimately bound to it. Diagnosis depends on the existence of classes that are ever shifting in their meaning, definitions, and relationships, as well as their persistence and usefulness. Classification is the process concerned with the setting up of classes, together with their changes and interrelationships. The classes, once established, are then available for the diagnostic process. In historical perspective, the classes are constantly shifting. The shifts, and the factors that brought them about, are a part of the study of classification. We must, therefore, turn from the diagnostic process and take up the correlative subject of classification.

# CHAPTER 5

## Classification

*Diagnosis takes place when someone makes a choice* among a series of classes. The series must have at least two members, but there is no upper limit. Then we have the problem: how do the classes get formed?

Classification depends on the perception of similarity, and whenever we perceive a similarity we deal with a class. A red brick and a red flower may not have much in common, but they do share the quality that we recognize and call "red." The important feature is not similarity-in-general but a similarity-in-at-least-one-particular, and this particular we call a "property." In all classes the members share some property. Conversely, if entities share a property, then they fall into some class. Adjectives and nouns indicate common classes of everyday speech.

Classification often has a highly practical function. When objects are suitably arranged, they are easy to find again. Furthermore, new objects can be placed into relation with those which have already been arranged. An obvious example is a library card-catalogue. The usefulness of classification must not blind us to another and quite different value, concerned with insight and understanding. For certain problems, classification supposedly provides not merely a useful tool but a fundamental insight into nature, reflecting the way things actually *are*. Classification would mirror reality. In such circumstances we *discover* the arrangement rather than create it.

There are thus two kinds of classification. The one, like the library catalogue, is arbitrary, and we ordinarily call it artificial. The other, however, is not arbitrary but depends on the "natural" order of things. Nature's order is not capricious. Its phenomena do not depend on human interest or convenience. The phenomena are *there*; they are organized, not random. Supposedly, through a "proper" classification, the investigator could discover the true organization of nature. This mode we call natural classification. The artificial arrangement has to do only with usefulness and convenience, natural classification with reality and truth. Both of these modes have played an extremely important part in the history of science and medicine. I want to take up three separate areas wherein the process of classification is important.

I

*Stamp Collecting: Artificial Classification*

A child starting to collect stamps might, if very young, paste all his specimens into a book, quite at random. He imposes no order upon them. If more mature, he will arrange them systematically in an album with a classification already prearranged: countries of origin, year of issue, and denomination. Then, in actual practice all he need do is decide whether this or that stamp belongs in this or that space. As we have seen, this constitutes the process of diagnosis.

Formal classification, which goes back to antiquity, has developed a special nomenclature, with terms such as class, order, genus, species, and variety (with additional terms as needed). This may sound strange in relation to stamp collecting, but use of these terms will enable us to compare the different examples and their special problems. The successive divisions proceed from the more general and more inclusive to the more specific and less inclusive. Each class "contains"—in a logical sense— the next succeeding.

The terms "genus" and "species" have a special importance. In its broadest sense, genus is any group within which there are subordinate groups. The genus has certain distinguishing marks, borne by every member within that class. The members, however, differ among themselves in other respects. They may be divided into coordinate sub-groups called species. Each species, in turn, may be capable of further subdivision, according to characteristic marks. In such a case each species becomes a genus in turn, with its own species. In this usage, genus and species indicate only the more general and the less general, as seen in the derivative terms "generic" and "specific."

The conventional stamp album shows an artificial classification with certain clear practical advantages. All stamps are well systematized, and any single stamp can readily be brought into relation with the others. Nevertheless, this particular mode of classification depends on certain interests and goals. If we have different interests and goals, then a different classification can be far more useful.

We might, for example, classify stamps according to the subject matter—animal stamps in one genus, landscapes in another, portraits in another. Animal stamps could be divided into mammals, fish, insects, and the like; landscapes into mountain, ocean, desert, and forest. An unsorted aggregate of postage stamps remains equally receptive to any of these classifications, none of which reflects any special reality.

There are, however, certain logical values that might apply. One classification can be more rigorous and can better avoid ambiguity or confusion. If a stamp shows a monkey in a forest, would this stamp be placed in the group *landscape* or the group *animal*? Obviously, it could go into either. Where such a possibility exists, logicians say that the divisions are not mutually exclusive. There are many such formal desiderata that characterize logical classification, but for details I would refer the reader to any textbook of formal logic.

For postage stamps or for any aggregate of other objects, there is no a priori limit to the number of artificial classifications that we might propound. Each will have certain advantages within the context for which it was designed, but may have disadvantages when construed in a different context but not in another. Usefulness is a major consideration, but we must always query, "useful for whom and under what condition?"

## II

### Classification of Plants

Among plants, discrimination arose from highly practical needs: early man had to distinguish the plants that could serve as food from those which could not. He also found that certain plants could satisfy other needs, such as clothing and shelter. And, furthermore, he learned through experience that some plants might cure or at least alleviate disease.

But, in addition to the practical functions, there were theoretical aspects to botany. The plant kingdom formed a major aspect of nature, whose study represented science. In science, however, the goal lay not in any practical advantages but rather in knowledge, considered as valuable for its own sake alone. The primary aim of science is understanding, not use. Any usefulness that might supervene would be an unexpected benefit.

Observers fully appreciated that plants were divisible into kinds, and that these kinds had some sort of relationship. Similarities were not random but suggested an underlying pattern. A radish and a carrot had distinct resemblances to each other, and both of them obviously differed from a grape or an olive. There seemed to be large groupings and then smaller groupings, and each class thus set up would have similarities and differences to other groups. Formal classification tried to organize the many individual groups into an orderly system.

Theophrastus (ca. 373-287 B.C.) was the first great systematic writer on botany. In his scheme of classification he made a primary division into trees, shrubs, and herbs, with further subdivisions into the cultivated and the wild, the flowering and the flowerless, the deciduous and the evergreen. He was a keen observer and was familiar, for example, with the difference between monocotyledons and dicotyledons, between roots and rhizomes. He knew that some flowers lacked petals and he discerned many fine differences in the relationships of the flower parts. His classification, however, did not rest on such fine distinctions and, indeed, some two thousand years had to pass before features such as these would play a role in formal classification. His own scheme of division depended on rather crude separations.

Botany as a branch of science did not flourish as much as did the more practical aspects. Dioscorides, active in the first century A.D., had a definitely practical bent, for he took account of function and as his primary division classified plants into the aromatic, the culinary, and the medicinal. To him we owe the first illustrated manuals of botany, the herbals, and their special medical orientation.

In contrast to this medical usefulness, the purely scientific interest in botany declined during the Middle Ages. During the Renaissance, however, an impetus to increased systematic study arose from several interconnected sources. Geographical explorations brought to the attention of scholars vast numbers of hitherto unknown plants that had to be integrated with existing knowledge. Curiosity became sharper. With an enhanced empirical attitude and an overall intellectual ferment, the 16th- and 17th-century workers paid much more attention to the detailed structure of plants. Early in the 17th century some 6,000 plants had been described, and the number increased enormously over the next century. Only an improved classification could bring order into this great variety.

There were thus two main currents in botany, the practical and the theoretical or scientific. For the practical aspects I am concerned only with the medicinal virtues and for the scientific currents, only with taxonomy. There were certain connecting links between the two. Many of the outstanding botanists were physicians or apothecaries. In the 16th century the herbal was the chief form of publication in botany, and herbals, originally, had a largely medical orientation and a practical function—to make available the information of medical interest. The herbal became the meeting place for the divergent currents that I call the medical and the taxonomic.

Those aspects of botany which described the medical use of plants were ultimately gathered into the special texts known as pharmacopeas, and the herbals became texts of systematic botany or taxonomy. The separation, dictated by many factors, took place gradually, but eventually the practical and the theoretical aspects, having separated, went their separate ways.

The transformation of the herbal into a text of systematic botany was punctuated by many efforts to achieve an orderly arrangement, to find principles of classification that would not only apply to all the known plants and accommodate new ones, but at the same time permit ready identification of individual specimens. Such efforts progressed slowly and with many confusing twists.

As the pharmacopea developed into a special form of scientific literature, and pharmacology into a distinct discipline, the therapeutic aspect of botany becomes oblique to our present problem. Our concern lies with the relationship between the classification of plants and the classification of diseases. This latter subject is known technically as nosology.

The problems of classifying diseases has intimate relations with the classification of plants. The crucial point of contact was the year 1676, for in that year Thomas Sydenham advocated the botanical method in the study of diseases. Sydenham wrote a much-quoted paragraph that led directly to the eventual growth of nosology: "It is necessary that all diseases be reduced to definite and certain *species*, and that, with the same care which we see exhibited by botanists in their phytologies; since it happens, at present, that many diseases, although included in the same genus, mentioned with a common nomenclature, and resembling one another in several symptoms, are, notwithstanding, different in their natures, and require a different medical treatment."[1]

The passage may seem a little murky at first glance, but it becomes clearer when we appreciate the status of botany at that time, and the parallelism Sydenham drew between diseases and plants. We must, furthermore, keep in mind the date at which he wrote, for the greatest progress in botanical taxonomy came later, especially from the work of Linnaeus in the next century.

The major problem was that of relationship: what things go together? No matter where we look, we will find both similarities and differences. On the basis of similarities we can place objects into distinct groups that bear certain relations to each other. At the same time some groups are more comprehensive than others. We have already mentioned this organization into genus and species when we discussed postage stamps in the preceding section. But in botany the identification of genus and species is more difficult and rests upon the insight of the individual. Similarities may be so numerous that the differences escape notice; or, conversely, there may be such vast differences that the similarities are not appreciated. The history of botanic taxonomy is, in a sense, the perception of similarities and differences, expressed as genera and species.

From the standpoint of logic, the first perception would be the recognition of discrete *kinds* of plants—there are oak trees, for example, and thistles, and roses, and they are not confused. But within any of these kinds that we call genera, how many subordinate kinds can we perceive, and how do we identify them? Conrad Gesner (1516-1565) declared: "There are scarcely any plants that constitute a genus which may not be divided into two or more species. The ancients described one species of gentian; I know of ten or more."[2] Gentian is a class that we can, if we want, call a genus. Into how many subordinate classes should it be divided?

The answer, of course, depends on the care with which we examine the different examples, the precision of our observations, and the insight with which we decide that *these* distinctions are important and indicate a separate class, while *those* differences are less important and come within the limits of expected variation. The problem that constantly bedevils taxonomists— when are we dealing with varieties and when with separate species?—existed in the 16th century just as much as in the 20th. To approach the problem we must describe carefully, note similarities and differences, evaluate them, and then decide on the groupings, whether superordinate, coordinate, or subordinate. In this way we set up genera and species, families and classes.

This is what the botanists were doing with plants and what Sydenham wanted the physicians to do with diseases. The first requisite was observation and description. The naturalists described plants; Sydenham wanted physicians to describe diseases with the same degree of care.

The botanists who described plants found many physical features to observe, and the great problem, as we shall see shortly, was to decide which features could serve as the basis for discrimination. In diseases the physician could attend to symptoms that, as I have insisted, meant any manifestations of the disease. The disease is recognizable through its symptoms in the same way that a plant is recognizable by its features.

For diseases Sydenham sought a relationship between genus and species and a parallelism to botanical classification. "We all know that the term *thistle* is applied to a variety of plants; nevertheless, he would be a careless botanist, indeed, who contented himself with the general description of a *thistle*; who only exhibited the marks by which the class was identified; who neglected the proper and peculiar signs of the species, and who overlooked the characters by which they were distinguished from each other. On the same principle, it is not enough for a writer to merely note down the common phenomena of some multiform disease. . . ."[3] He was saying, in effect, that among diseases the physician must identify the genus and then search for characters that would distinguish the species.

The relationship between plants and diseases Sydenham expressed in a further well-known passage. "Nature, in the production of disease, is uniform and consistent; so much so, that for the same disease in different persons the symptoms are for the most part the same; and the selfsame phenomena that you would observe in the sickness of a Socrates you would observe in the sickness of a simpleton. Just so the universal characters of a plant are extended to every individual of the species; and whoever (I speak in the way of illustration) should accurately describe the colour, the taste, the smell, the figure, &c., of one single violet, would find that his description held good, there or thereabouts, for all the violets of that particular species upon the face of the earth."[4]

Since Sydenham drew comparisons between botany and medicine, we must examine the state of botanical classification *at the time that he wrote*. We can appropriately ask, "How much success had the botanists achieved in their classifications?" Clearly, Sydenham thought that they had been quite successful, for otherwise he would not have recommended the application of botanical methods to medicine.

Many identifications are quite simple: we do not need a formal discipline to distinguish an onion from a marigold. These would represent easily recognizable genera. Difficulties arise when we try to show the relationship of different genera to each other or to break down the genera into species, or to group genera into larger and more comprehensive classes. What sort of criteria can serve as the principles of relationship, or of division, or of aggregation? Details of the steps whereby the principles gradually became more refined belong in technical histories of botany, but a few features we may note here.

There were several interlocking lines of development. One important trend was the increasing use of a so-called artificial principle of classification. Some single feature or small cluster of features would serve as the basis on which the various plants could be divided. For example, the properties of the leaf, or the character of the fruit or the seed, or particular aspects of the corolla, might serve as criteria whereby subordinate groups could be set up. These arbitrary criteria might, however, bring into relation classes that otherwise were markedly divergent, that "agreed in at least a single character . . . though they differed in almost everything else."[5]

An artificial classification, then, rests on some predetermined feature. It contrasts with the so-called natural classification that tries to take the plants as a whole, consider all the features as they exist in nature, and seek the overall similarities. Since "all" is impossible to describe, the natural mode of classification necessarily requires a great many similar features to establish the groupings.

A further important feature in the history of botany is the development of a binomial nomenclature, whereby any member of the plant kingdom receives two names, one indicating the genus, and the other, by providing some sort of a differential feature, indicating the species. Gaspard Bauhin (1560-1624) is generally credited with establishing this procedure, although suggestions of binomial designation occur earlier.

There was thus a trend toward precision, minute observation, and careful discrimination, within the limits of available knowl-

edge. Yet, in the 17th century the concepts of botanical classification were far too fluid and a flora—still called an herbal—
would show a division that we today would call a hodgepodge,
confusing many families that we consider entirely distinct.

At this point it is important to restrict ourselves to the texts
prior to Sydenham's 1676 publication, for only then can we
appreciate the factors that influenced his thought. One of the
most striking and valuable of these texts is John Parkinson,
*Theatrum Botanicum: The Theatre of Plants, or, an Herbal of
Large Extent.*[6] This huge folio, excellently illustrated, has 17
subdivisions, designated as "tribes." Each tribe circumscribes a
particular major grouping. The titles, indicating the subject
matter, help us to understand the attitudes of the era. I list all
17 tribes, with the original spelling.

These are Parkinson's tribes: 1. Sweete smelling Plants; 2.
Purging Plants; 3. Venemous, Sleepy, and Hurtfull Plants, and
their Counterpoysons; 4. Saxifrages or Breakestone Plants; 5.
Vulnerary or Wound Herbes; 6. Cooling and Succory-like
Herbes; 7. Hot and sharpe biting Plants; 8. Umbelliferous
Plants; 9. Thistles and Thorny Plants; 10. Fearns and Capillary
Herbes; 11. Pulses; 12. Cornes; 13. Grasses, Rushes and
Reades; 14. Marsh, Water, and Sea Plants, and Mosses and
Mushromes; 15. The Unordered Tribe; 16. Trees and Shrubbes;
17. Strange and Outlandish Plants.

Some authors deride a table of contents such as this as showing a lack of "scientific" acumen. Yet since Parkinson's book
(and others like it) has particular importance for the study of
nosology, we should note what it actually does and does not do.

For one thing, it illustrates the difference between enumeration and classification. Parkinson had made certain arbitrary
groupings, each of which gathers together the plants that show
some particular property. We can make a comparison. Suppose,
in a given community, we list all the people who own automo-
biles. We would then have a group with one particular feature
in common, although they would differ in other respects. Then
suppose we made another list, of persons who graduated from
college, and still another, of persons over six feet tall. *In each*

*list* the members would have at least one factor in common. Each list, however, was compiled for a different purpose. One has to do with vehicular property, another with education, and the third with physical appearance. Any individual might appear in one, two, or three of the lists, but some members of the community might appear in none.

Formal logic would tell us that this is a bad classification, for the separate groups do not in the aggregate include all the persons in the community, and as separate categories they permit overlap. They represent enumerations. A classification should make clear the way that the separate groupings relate to each other, as superordinate, coordinate, or subordinate. The three lists do not bear to each other any of these relationships. Vehicular property, education, and stature are quite unrelated or, if they are related, the connection is not made clear.

So it is with Parkinson's arrangement of the 17 listings. Some have to do with medicinal virtues: all the plants in one listing have a laxative quality, while in another grouping all act as sedatives. Other categories indicate the habitat: the members may grow in marshes or in a watery environment. Other categories, such as grasses or ferns, show a distinctive morphology. One class distinguishes plants that are woody: the trees and shrubs. Another includes plants that do not fit into any of the other groups: the "unordered" individuals. The last tribe has, as its unifying common feature, that the members are all strange and bizarre.

The principles underlying the enumeration—e.g., the medicinal properties or manner of growth or mophology—are as disparate as the categories of vehicular property, education, or physical appearance. Furthermore, there is nothing exclusive about the listings. A mushroom can be poisonous and shrubs and trees can be sweet-smelling.

Nevertheless, we must recognize a certain merit: each listing can serve a useful function. The physician who wants to learn about purgatives or sedatives or poisons knows where to turn, and so too does the farmer who is curious about grasses, "cornes," and "pulses." The individual sections contain a great

deal of information and describe, often quite well, many different specimens. The plants, Parkinson said, were "Distributed
into sundry Classes or Tribes, for the/ more easie knowledge of
the many Herbes of one nature/ and property. . . ."[7]

The listings do not conform to the divisions of orders, families, and genera that we use today. Thus, in Parkinson's tribe
of purgative plants there are listed aloes and yucca, belonging
to the lily family; dock and rhubarb, members of the buckwheat
family; colocynth, in the gourd family; and scammony in the
morning glory family. Among the purgatives he listed 66 kinds
of plants, or genera (many of which had several species). But,
while they represented many different botanical families, they
had in common the important feature that they all acted as purgatives.

I have discussed Parkinson at some length for two reasons.
He compiled a major work of botany, important at the time
when Sydenham recommended that physicians should follow the
example of botanists. Second, Parkinson's actual presentation is
extremely relevant to the classification of diseases that appeared
in the 18th century.

As Arber declared, botanical science tries to arrange plants
"according to the affinities which they present when considered
in themselves, and not in relation to man."[8] Parkinson has done
this only to a limited degree. The *Theatrum* did serve a practical
function; it was useful in many different contexts, but it did not
promote any comprehensive understanding of the plant kingdom. In the search for an ever-widening, ever-more-compre-
hensive unity, Parkinson has not achieved success.

After Sydenham's death (1689) John Ray (1627-1705) and
Joseph Tournefort (1656-1708) made major contributions, but
the most important figure in taxonomy was Carl Linné, or Linnaeus (1707-1778), the subject of an enormous critical and historical literature.[9] He described vast numbers of plants, integrated many of the botanical advances of the earlier periods, and
set new procedural standards. He devised a highly logical system of classification—the so-called sexual system, whose details,
however, we do not need to discuss here.

The achievement of Linnaeus formed the high point of the so-called artificial systems that depend on arbitrary criteria, but, as he himself fully realized, his system did not pay adequate attention to the "natural affinities." According to modern theory, the basis for a natural system of classification rests on the concept of common ancestry, and requires study and comparison of a large number of properties, rather than merely one or two. The various criticisms of Linnaeus, and the development of further classificatory schemata, will be found in histories of botany.

Linnaeus, who was a physician, classified not only plants but also animals and diseases. In 1763 he published a small volume, *Genera Morborum*, in which he arranged and described 325 different *kinds* of disease, or genera. In the study of disease, however, he was far less important than his contemporary, also a physician, Francois Boissier de Sauvages de la Croix (1706-1767), who published a preliminary study of nosology in 1734 and a monumental work in 1763.[10]

### III

*Eighteenth-Century Nosology*

Sydenham's plea had not found an immediate response, and many years had to pass before his vision became translated into concrete performance. In the half century or so after his death, there developed a sense of unrest among empirically minded physicians. In 1733 a Scottish physician expressed great dissatisfaction with the confusion then prevalent in medicine:

"It has been the misfortune of this art to be loaded with such numbers of names to each disease, and such minute and subtile distinctions of them, by which a beginner, on viewing a catalog of distempers in some of the systematick writers, will be apt to imagine that each name denotes a disease very different from any other . . . ; whereas if the matter was duly considered, it would appear that these numerous lists might be much abridged, by reducing many diseases to the same class or general head." No two diseases, he went on, are "strictly parallel in every circumstance," but every case should not therefore have a new name. The proper course was "to set aside all the smaller differences and accidental circumstances, and to search out that which is of most consequence in any disease. . . ."[11]

Here was an expressed desire for systematization, to bring order into multiplicity. At the very time that this was being written in Scotland, the young French physician Boissier de Sauvages was undertaking exactly such a task. His first book, published in 1734, led eventually to the great and definitive text of 1763, and there followed a succession of other nosologies, well into the 19th century.[12]

Sauvages did indeed provide an orderly classification of diseases in botanical fashion, as Sydenham had recommended. In the preface of this early work he set forth some fundamental principles. He accepted the sharp distinction between the theory of medicine and its practice that Baglivi had already emphasized. Theory rested on causes, but *causes could not serve as a basis for classification*. Causes were matters of inference, not direct observation, and usually comprised hypothetical and imaginary entities.[13]

Today we are so wedded to the importance of cause in the classification of disease that we find difficulty in grasping the force of Sauvages' comment. But if we reflect on causes that are admittedly hypothetical, his position becomes quite acceptable. Would we today classify behavior disorders according to the presence or absence of an inferiority complex? Or an inadequate superego? These concepts are indeed hypotheses to explain some behavior patterns, but they could never serve as basis for a reliable classification. In the 18th century the causes of most diseases were largely hypothetical, often analogous to the inferiority complex.

Like Sydenham, Sauvages emphasized the need for an adequate natural history of diseases that would indicate their character, manner of origin and termination, and mode of treatment. The prodigious number and variety of diseases resembled the variety and number of plants. Medicine should reduce the natural history of diseases to classes, genera, and species, as did botany. In attempting this task Sauvages had a practical goal.

He wanted to arrange and characterize diseases so that their recognition was simple and assured. This was possible only if he attended to phenomena that could be directly observed. And this, in turn, required a classification by *symptoms*, and by symptoms alone.[14]

A symptom, as we have already seen, was any observable manifestation of disease. However, since for any given disease the symptoms were both multiple and variable, a sound classification could rest only on those phenomena which were *essential* and *constant*. These are the key words. The symptoms that would permit the classification of disease must be neither variable in their occurrence nor accidental (in the Aristotelian sense) in their nature.

A disease, then, for Sauvages, was an entity that manifests itself by characteristic and constant disturbances that the physician can perceive directly. The causes of disease, whether hypothetical, like acrids, or more concrete, like worms, or intermediate, like miasmas, could not serve as the basis for classification.

Sauvages' goal was mainly practical. He wanted not to advance theoretical medicine but to make it easy for a student or physician to identify any disease that affected a patient. A sound classification, he felt, would achieve this aim. He paid lip service to logical requirements. He thought that the aggregate of classes should contain all the diseases and that no disease should belong to more than one class. These two requirements comprise the well-known desideratum, "jointly exhaustive and mutually exclusive." Furthermore, as a concession to students, the number of primary classes should be small and should presuppose only a minimum knowledge of anatomy and physiology.

In this early work Sauvages offered 10 primary classes that differ somewhat from the arrangement in his *Nosologia* of 1763. Our further discussion will derive from this later work. The early book is especially important for the methodology, markedly expanded in the mature work published almost thirty years later.

For Sauvages the most general symptoms would define the

most general categories of disease and he could then proceed in graduated stages to the more specific. Sauvages pointed to 10 entirely general manifestations to identify the broadest groupings or *classes*. Each class had some dominant feature—e.g., fever, or inflammation, or spasm, or respiratory difficulty, or pain, or weakness.

Each of the 10 superordinate *classes* was further subdivided into several subordinate *orders*, according to some discriminating feature. The class of weakness, for example, was subdivided according to the function affected. (The term "weakness" included all degrees of diminished function up to and including complete loss.) One subdivision would involve the diminution of sensation; another, of voluntary movement; another, of appetites; another, of "vital forces"; and a final group, diminution or loss of all functions, as would occur in apoplexy or coma.

Each *order* was further subdivided into kinds or *genera*, coordinate with each other. In the order, loss of voluntary movement, Sauvages distinguished among the genera muteness, or the inability to articulate words; aphonia, the inability to make any vocal sounds at all; stuttering, the inability to pronounce some syllables. These genera, covering various defects in the voice, were coordinate with other kinds of weakness that affected muscles of the limbs and trunk—e.g., paralysis, the diminished power to move a limb; hemiplegia, the weakness of one whole side of the body; and paraplegia, the weakness or paralysis of the lower extremities.

Each *genus* was subdivided into *species* that represented individual diseases. Thus, under hemiplegia Sauvages listed 14 species. One he called scrofulous; another, traumatic; another, epileptic; another, a hemiplegia occurring in workers in lead mines.

The ultimate subjects of the classification were the individual diseases. How did he know what to classify? The answer for him is exactly the same as it would be for us today—he relied partly on what he himself had observed, but more on what he had read in the literature. We today are so engulfed in a tidal wave of case reports that we do not appreciate the vast amount of medical literature existing in the 18th century. Sauvages took his species—the individual unit-diseases—from the voluminous writings of both contemporary and earlier physicians. There were the massive tomes of the 17th-century writers; the "centuries" and other case reports of the 18th-century physicians; the compendia of autopsy reports; the monographs on individual diseases; and an already voluminous periodical literature. Whatever anyone had described as a disease, Sauvages tended to accept as a species.

Unfortunately, the same condition might be variously reported under different names (as frequently happens today). Reports would vary in degree of completeness and the reliability of the original observer (just as happens today). Sauvages had no way to weed out duplication or determine accuracy. If we ask, then, what it was that Sauvages was classifying, we must answer: *he was classifying the conditions that other physicians had called diseases*. His great defect was not so much in his methodology as in his lack of critical sense. He was credulous. Many of his species represent single cases reported in extremely inadequate detail. The poorly reported cases and the well-reported cases were accepted equally. For this reason many of the 14 species of hemiplegia are quite unintelligible today.

Sauvages was classifying diseases, but his ideas of disease differed from ours. I suggest, however, that the differences were quantitative rather than qualitative. The differential features, unfortunately, were inadequate in number and precision; he did not have enough data to make rigorous distinctions; he lacked a detailed natural history and sharp discriminatory traits. In his survey he relied largely on hearsay evidence, much of it of doubtful validity. He needed more and better evidence. In time this did come into being, along two lines: improved observation increased the number of recognized symptoms; and research broadened the *meaning* of these symptoms and the relationships into which they entered (the "knowledge-about" to which I refer in other chapters). Physiology provided significance to phenomena that otherwise would have escaped notice. So too with the data and concepts of pathology and chemistry and other relevant sciences. Thanks to these basic sciences, new phenomena were observed, acquired meaning, and then led to greater precision in discriminating diseases.

Historically, an important step in this process came from increased clinico-pathological correlations. Individual symptoms acquired greater meaning when they were correlated with pathological changes. And this increased knowledge, in turn, allowed sharper clinical distinctions. The correlation of symptoms with structural changes permitted discrimination among conditions that had previously seemed uniform.

Progress in medicine, I maintain, comes from increased discrimination. Whereas Sauvages and his 18th-century colleagues had to rely on their unaided senses; physicians in the 19th century had the advantage of instruments that led to more precise discrimination. And these, in turn, often led to the identification of new disease entities. At the same time the basic sciences were expanding the meaning of symptoms. The more symptoms that came to the attention of the physician, and the richer their meaning, the more accurate would be his discriminations and the more precise the disease entity.

Sauvages had a limited view of the disease entity, and the data on which he relied proved to be weak reeds indeed. His great difficulty was not in depending on symptoms for his classification, but in not having enough symptoms to depend on. They were not sharp enough, or numerous enough, to provide stability to his groupings. Of course, when he contrived his system he did not know its inadequacies. These came to light as part of medical progress. Our present-day failure to appreciate what he was trying to do comes largely from our failure to understand the meaning of "symptom" in the 18th century, and our modern lamentable confusion between symptoms and signs.

Sauvages intended his classification for practical use (in addition to theoretical enlightenment). To indicate the way a physician could identify the disease from which the patient was suffering, he gave a concrete example. Suppose, he said, we find a woman stretched out on the ground, unconscious, with no power of voluntary movement. Whoever knows the classes of disease will immediately recognize that she comes under *class* 6 (weaknesses), and the *order*, comatose conditions. The different genera in this order each have its distinguishing feature by which it can be discriminated from all the others. By comparing the features observed in the patient with the features that define the different genera, the physician will quickly come to the *genus* apoplexy. Then he must find the particular species—the precise niche. Does the apoplexy arise from trauma or plethora or cachexia, or any of the other delimited types? The physician discovers these aspects by physical examination, by investigating the circumstances, and by skillful questioning of the bystanders.[15]

In his text, emphasis on symptoms is in no way inconsistent with a concern with causes. On knowledge of cause depend the full *understanding* of the condition and the appropriate therapy. However, the point at issue is, how best to provide a classification? Sauvages insisted repeatedly, and with complete justification, that the only way to achieve a sound classification was *through what the physician could actually observe*. And this meant symptoms. From the observation of symptoms the physician could then *infer* the responsible agent and institute proper treatment.

In this process the symptoms would serve as *signs* that pointed toward the cause. Signs had to be interpreted, and this involved conjecture. Classification, however, must depend not on conjecture but on sound definition; and definition, to be useful, must contain only those essential elements which can be constantly observed. Factors that are conjectured (as well as inconstant or trivial) do not make a satisfactory definition, and therefore have no place in making a classification.

## IV

### Present-Day Nosology

Although Sauvages used a terminology that seems strange to us, nevertheless his methodology is in essence the same that we use today, although in a somewhat different context. We no longer use the taxonomic terms classes, orders, genera, and species and we classify disease on a rather different framework. But when we try to identify a disease we use the same method that he advocated.

We can have more sympathy if we regard Sauvages' ten classes not as entities but only as organizing principles whereby we reduce into manageable order the immense complexity of symptoms. We today are constantly using particular symptoms as guides for further analysis. If, for example, we find that a patient has high blood pressure, we immediately have a major category within which we can carry out a systematic study.

Unfortunately, today we are obsessed with the notion of cause and we do not bother to sort out the confusion inherent in this term. Instead of asking, "What are the different *causes* of hypertension?" Sauvages would properly have asked, "How many different *kinds* of hypertension are there?"

In the 18th century hypertension was unknown. Assume, however, that Sauvages were living today. He would want to know, "How can we distinguish one kind of hypertension from another?" He might, for example, separate off a group where the primary disturbance is in the kidney, and then he would distinguish further sub-groups of kidney disease, such as glomerulonephritis or diabetic nephropathy. In other kinds of hypertension the endocrine glands seem to be involved; in other groups, drugs or toxic agents. In still others there are emotional disturbances. And on and on and on, with many distinguishable *kinds* of hypertension.

If Sauvages were alive today, he would have had a splendid time trying to place the different kinds in an orderly arrangement, with definite relations to each other, and he would have called the different groupings by the appropriate taxonomic name of class, order, genus, and species. We today would not think of doing this, but we might make up a table, and distinguish the various headings by roman numerals, capital letters, arabic numerals, lower-case letters (and, if further organization were needed, by Greek letters or the use of primes and double primes).[16]

Sauvages knew nothing about hormonal assays, arteriograms,

or renal biopsies, or other such laboratory data. But, if he did, he would have regarded them as criteria to distinguish one group from another. If a renal biopsy, for example, showed certain microscopic changes, these would merely have comprised a *symptom* of the disease from which the patient suffered. Such a symptom would be comparable to an edema of the ankles or to changes in the eyegrounds. And, by observing enough of these manifestations, Sauvages would have found the correct *kind* of hypertension.

I have mentioned hypertension as a term around which we can categorize a wide range of conditions. High blood pressure is a striking symptom. It permits an easy organization into subordinate groups, all with a common feature. So too with the symptom jaundice, a feature that quickly attracts attention. When a physician today sees a patient with jaundice, he immediately starts thinking of the various "causes," uses certain procedures to eliminate some, rule in others, and finally zeroes in on the proper category. Sauvages, in the 18th century, did exactly the same thing, except that he looked for kinds rather than causes. In the *class* cachexias, he had as his sixth *order* the diseases in which there was a *change in color*. The *genera* included yellow jaundice, black jaundice, and red jaundice. (As a further kind of "depraved color," he included pallor, which we would call "anemia" but which he called "chlorosis.")

Among the different *species* of yellow jaundice Sauvages distinguished various disturbances of the liver, jaundice associated with poisons, with obstruction and calculi, with suppuration, with various types of fever, occasionally with pregnancy, and with plethora. He made his discriminations by features that he observed. Today, the physician who sees a patient with jaundice thinks of the different conditions in which jaundice is a symptom. Then, in systematic fashion, he tries to determine the particular disease from which the patient is suffering. The techniques are different, but the procedure is essentially the same as Sauvages recommended.

Sauvages was offering a framework for diagnosis, and a method by which the patient could be placed in the appropriate niche. His classes and groupings seem dreadfully confused to us, and his defining characteristics entirely inadequate as well as erroneous. But the lack of knowledge did not affect the methodology. He had neither the knowledge nor the tools to make sounder discriminations.

The modern textbook of medicine, with its vast array of diseases, offers a nosology in its table of contents. The various diseases must be placed in some sort of order. And the table of contents—as example we can take a modern text such as Beeson-McDermott—shows some of the problems that troubled Sauvages and still trouble physicians who try to bring order into medicine.

What diseases would be juxtaposed? And in what relationship? And according to what principle? The infectious diseases are quite easy, for there we can have an arrangement that we fondly consider etiological. We can take the major groups of microbiological agents—viruses, Rickettsias, bacteria, spirochetes, fungi, protozoa, metazoa—and let each serve as the distinguishing mark for major groups of diseases. Each group can then be divided in turn according to the genus of organism—myxoviruses, enteroviruses, and so on; Streptococcus, Clostridium, Salmonella, and so on; Plasmodium, Trypanosoma, and the like. Sub-subgroups can be inserted as desired. We can readily classify a couple of hundred distinct diseases in this way, allegedly by cause.

But then the difficulties start. How to classify other diseases? What major overall groupings should be used? We can set up various functional systems: locomotive, nervous, respiratory, cardiovascular, renal, digestive, hematopoietic. Some diseases, however, seem to affect the body much more widely, such as diseases of metabolism, immune diseases, hereditary diseases.

Within any single major division the individual conditions are held together by a sound unifying principle, in the same way as were the plants within each division of Parkinson's *Theatrum Botanicum*. But the relation of one major grouping to another is no more logical than was Parkinson's. Moreover, any given disease is not restricted to a single category. Should an infection of the kidney come under infectious diseases or renal diseases, or both?

Fortunately, it doesn't really matter. The modern editors, fully aware of the difficulties, are not trying to classify diseases in order to satisfy the strict canons of logic. They are trying to present the data of medicine in a way that would be maximally useful for medical practitioners and students—just as did Sauvages. Classifications are made for use. If there is a conflict between use and logic, then logic goes out the window.

We find a good brief summary of general principles in the *Manual of the International Statistical Classification of Diseases, Injuries, and Causes of Death* (1977): "A classification of diseases may be defined as a system of categories to which morbid entities are assigned according to some established criteria. There are many possible choices for these criteria . . . many axes of classification and the particular axis selected will be determined by the interest of the investigator. . . . The goal of this particular classification was "storage, retrieval and tabulation of data."[17] Sauvages, and Beeson and McDermott, had quite different goals. Sometimes, however, the goals are not clearly defined, and then we run into special difficulty.

*DISEASE*

## CHAPTER 6

# Disease and Health

*If I pose the question*, "What is disease?" the answer will depend on whom I ask. There is the patient who has a disease, and the physician or healer who tries to cure him. There is also the scientist, who may or may not be a physician. In either case the scientist does not concern himself with the direct care of the patient but rather with the overall advancement of knowledge. The patient seeks relief, the physician tries to provide it, and the scientist seeks understanding.

Disease is an abstract term. Ordinarily we define an abstraction by studying the concrete examples and finding the property that they have in common. We can readily point to individual conditions such as pneumonia, gout, appendicitis, and hundreds of comparable states discussed in a textbook of medicine. These all differ one from the other. What is the uniting thread?

At first glance this common factor might seem quite easy to find: all we need do is examine the properties of the various states regarded as diseases and note what they have in common. But actually this will not work. We cannot lay out for examination a whole series of separate states identified as diseases unless we know in advance what it is that makes them diseases. Is alcoholism a disease, or addiction to tobacco, or homosexuality? If we say "yes," then we have already implied a particular definition. If, on the other hand, we say "no," then we automtically have a different definition. No one, perhaps, will disagree about pneumonia or appendicitis, but there is ample disagreement about, say, alcoholism. Before we can list a number of conditions to find out what they have in common, we must agree on which ones we are going to put in that list. And, obviously, before we do that, we must have in mind some criteria that determine our selection. And that is precisely what we are trying to find—the criteria by which we identify a disease. And this necessarily involves the relation of disease to health.

Here we run into a further complication. In 1980 alcoholism might or might not be considered a disease, but in 1880 there was no problem at all: alcoholism was not a disease but a moral failure. In 1780 fever was considered a disease; in 1980 it is regarded not as a disease at all but as a symptom. If we try to frame a definition, should we restrict ourselves to the views of the past ten years, or should we take into account what people thought one hundred or two hundred or five hundred years ago?

I

*Some Traditional Views*

We can start our analysis by considering some traditional views that are still highly influential. I will go no farther back than the 17th century. At that time the Galenic concepts still dominated medical theory. The physicians who maintained these views, with more or less divergence from Galen, I have called neogalenists, of whom Daniel Sennert (1572-1637) is an excellent example. In his voluminous writings he made many references to health and disease, regarded as opposite. A satisfactory definition for one would automatically establish the definition of the other.[1]

The notions of health or disease revolved around the concept of nature, a term both complex and vague. Nature meant, among other things the way things were—the aggregate of existence as we find it. This is a descriptive sense. By studying nature we learn what actually exists and in what proportion, not, of course, in any statistical sense but only by vague intuition.

There was also a second sense to the term "nature," namely, the way things ought to be. Today the words "normal" and "norm" share this dual sense. Normal has a descriptive force, made more effective by actual enumeration and calculation. The word "norm" conveys in part the idea of a standard or type or model, and implies something desirable, or what ought to exist.

In the Galenic tradition, "according to nature" meant something both prevalent and desirable. "Contrary to nature" was abnormal and undesirable. The natural implied a standard to which things ought to conform. A certain amount of leeway was acceptable, but the limits of the permissible deviations were not at all clear.

In matters of health the important variable was function or performance. Sennert declared: "All men consider themselves healthy when, through the help of the bodily parts, they are able to perform the functions according to nature, and necessary for life, without any impairment (*vitio*) or hindrance. By general agreement those persons are considered sick who cannot perform those activities, or at least, not without impairment." To be healthy a man need not actually perform the actions but he must be capable of doing so.[2]

From the definition of health we can easily reach a knowledge of disease. "Disease is most correctly defined as the inability of performing functions in a natural fashion." And just as healthy people are capable of acting according to nature, "those persons are properly called sick who are incapable of performing those functions." As a slight variant he declared, disease is "a constitution or disposition *praeter naturam*, that impairs activity. . . . A disease is a disposition of the bodily parts that is defective and diverges from the natural state, whereby the persons are rendered incapable and unsuitable for performing the functions naturally (*actiones naturales*)." Disease consisted of disability, judged by what was considered natural.[3]

By the late 17th century the intellectual climate was changing, and the Galenic ideas gave way to the mechanical philosophy wherein the phenomena of the living body were thought to follow the laws of mechanics, which governed particles in motion. Friedrich Hoffmann (1660-1742), who enthusiastically embraced the new philosophy, defined health in accord with the laws of mechanics: "the energetic action of both body and mind, depending on a proportionate and free motion of the solids and the fluids, and a due proportion of the blood and humors." What comprised the due proportion was not defined, but, whatever it was, the failure in that respect characterized disease. Disease, the opposite of health, consisted in "a great change and disturbance in the proportion and order of the motions," along with which there was "striking disturbance of secretions, excretions, and other functions of the living body."[4]

Hoffmann stressed a certain minimal level of disturbance before a condition could properly be called a disease. He made this clear through his choice of adjectives. The terms "great change" and "striking disturbance" tell us that minor alterations are not to be considered diseases. Presumably they were to be ignored.

Herman Boerhaave (1668-1738) offered further specifications: "The person who can perform the several actions proper to the human body with ease, pleasure, and a certain constancy, is said to be well; and that condition of the body is termed health. But if he either cannot perform those actions; or if he performs them but with difficulty, pain, and sudden weariness; he is then said to be ill: and that state of the body is called a disease." Here, as with Sennert, we have a renewed emphasis on function. In addition, Boerhaave specifically noted the subjective sense of pleasure in healthy functioning, and he indicated pain as a component of disease.[5]

He noted further that what in one person would constitute disease might in another person be consistent with health. Health, based on the idea of proportion, did not require equality. Individual differences were taken into account, so that in various people one or another humor might predominate, yet each person could be healthy according to his own temperament. The temperaments—i.e., the relative proportions of the humors—will differ one from the other, yet each may in its own way represent complete health. This concept, that large individual differences can nevertheless all fall within the category of health, is an important legacy of classical medicine.[6]

By the mid-18th century several features that distinguished health and disease were already defined in terms that are still important today. The formulations persisted without much change into the middle of the 19th century. By that time, however, there were already evident certain changes in the intellectual climate that placed health and disease in a new perspective, one that has been continuously changing until the present. The central feature is the distinction between the medical practitioner and the medical scientist. In an earlier period a distinction was not valid. All medical practitioners took care of patients; and some practitioners, in addition, helped to expand the theoretical basis of medicine. These were the medical scientists of their time. The scientist, through discovering new data and propounding generalizations and explanations, enlarges the frontiers of knowledge. Gifted practitioners expanded knowledge at the same time that they practiced medicine. As practitioners, they were concerned with particular patients and their care; as scientists, with generalizations, explanations, and theories.

When these two distinct activities were performed by the same physician, the concept of disease was patient-centered. But by the middle of the 19th century there was already evident a significant change—the medical sciences were separating from the actual care of the patient. Physiology, chemistry, and pathology, as emerging disciplines, claimed more and more allegiance of their devotees. Each of these subjects became a science in its own right and demanded highly specialized training. Professional pathologists, physiologists, and chemists no longer practiced clincial medicine to any extent, but attended to their laboratory disciplines.

There began an era of laboratory medicine, characterized by experimentation and the development of special technology. All this we may contrast with the earlier activities that I call observational medicine. Brilliant examples abounded in the early 19th century, when clinicians such as Laennec, Louis, Bretonneau, Hodgkin, Bright, Stokes, Adams, Addison, to name but a few, greatly expanded the frontiers of medicine through precise observation. For these men the post-mortem examination was a major tool, but experimentation was not a factor and new technologies were not involved. These clinicians gave us improved discrimination and greater understanding in medicine. But, while they furnished greater discrimination, they were not so successful in providing explanations. For this we must reach different levels of description and correlation.[7]

These deeper levels came about through the basic sciences in medicine—anatomy, physiology, chemistry, pathology, pharmacology—that could answer questions through experiments. The scientists could propound "laws that had explanatory value and could correlate their data with what was going on in the healthy and in the diseased.

Even though the medical scientists studied aspects of disease, their interest lay with the interrelations among the phenomena rather than with the immediate connection with the sick patient. There was a trend toward so-called "pure" science, the study of phenomena for their own sake. Any generalizations achieved thereby might indeed help in patient care, but the main interest lay in finding relationships, establishing their validity, and constructing explanatory theories. Pure science had its origins in disinterested curiosity.

The medical scientists were concerned with the questions, "What happens if . . . ?" or "What happens when . . . ?" With such questions in mind, the traditional distinctions between health and disease, between normal and abnormal, became blunted. The concept of disease tended to get submerged in the broader area, the interrelation of bodily functions under various conditions. Particular conditions would produce particular results. The discovery of the correlations was more important than the question as to whether this or that condition represented disease. Of primary concern was the question, "How do various changes in circumstances affect the structure or function?" and not "What changes should be called disease?" The biological sciences were concerned with the interaction between an organism (or its components) and its enviroment (both internal and external).

For the basic scientist the problem as to which reactions represent disease and which ones represent health is not truly relevant. On the other hand, the question holds primary interest for the physician, who takes care of patients. He must know what he is trying to cure, and what constitutes a cure. The basic scientist has no concern with these questions.

By the middle of the 19th century this attitude was beginning to make itself felt in the medical literature. In 1852, in a text entitled *Medical Logic*, we find the author saying: "What we are accustomed to call disease is but a peculiar change or process in the living organism, under the action of some of those influences from without, which affect the maintenance, loss and recovery of health; and these changes are a part—a very small one—of the great whole of nature."[8]

At the end of the 19th century Sir Clifford Albutt expressed this viewpoint somewhat more elegantly: "Disease is a state of a living organism, a balance of function more unstable than that which we call health; its causes may be imported, or the system may 'rock' from some implicit defect, but the disease itself is a perturbation which contains no elements essentially different from those of health, but *elments presented in a different and less useful order*."[9]

This emphasis on usefulness brings into consideration a special set of values. The scientist studies reactions. Some of these, deemed useful, refer to health; some, not useful, are labelled disease. But then we immediately face the problem: useful for whom and according to what criteria? Who determines whether or not the reactions are useful?

## II

In 1954 I published a paper entitled "What is Disease?"[10] in which I emphasized the role of social and cultural factors in identifying the disease state. Subsequently, the query, in its modern context, received a great deal of attention. The published viewpoints are quite diverse, and even a cursory examination would carry us far afield. While I indicate some of the important recent publications,[11] I will not attempt any critical analysis. In the present context I will rest content with presenting my own views.

No one will dispute the time-honored view that conditions (or reactions) that induce disability and may lead to death are properly called disease: pneumonia, cancer, gout, coronary occlusion, are representative entities of this group. But there are other conditions not so clear, in which the designation of disease may or may not be offered, according to the prevalent cultural pattern.

Sometimes, in a particular culture, bodily changes may be deliberately induced to bring about a state considered useful and desirable. Thus, at one period the Chinese bound the feet of certain female infants, to produce skeletal and muscular distortions—atrophy of the feet and hypertrophy of the buttocks—that supposedly made the girls sexually more attractive at puberty. A different culture, however, judges these young women to be crippled and diseased, rather than having specially desirable and highly valued characteristics. Comparably, some African tribes deliberately elongate the necks of female children. This they accomplish by placing an increasing number of rings around the neck, starting in early childhood. The resulting elongation was thought to enhance sexual attractiveness. However, the neck muscles become atrophic, so that if the rings are removed, the women are unable to hold up their heads. They may even die from angulation of the trachea. Our Western culture considers this an example of disease.

These two examples illustrate an artificially induced deformity that could be useful in certain environments, harmful in others. Western culture provides its own examples: e.g., during the 19th century, fashion demanded that women encase themselves in tightly laced corsets. These might produce an hour-glass deformity of the liver, the so-called corset liver mentioned in all the older textbooks of pathology.

Many other traits and reactions may or may not be considered disease, according to the prevalent cultural patterns. In certain eras and environments, trance states and even epileptic attacks may be regarded as a sign of divine afflatus. A different culture would regard the conditions as disease. In some political environments a leader may attract an enormous following and be considered highly charismatic; other cultures may regard him as suffering from paranoia or other dangerous abnormalities.

The particular interactions that lead to atrophy or hypertrophy, or the factors in convulsions, or the mental state called paranoia, we can regard as events in the world of science. Calling them disease or, conversely, refusing to call them disease, is a societal judgment. We cannot understand what we mean by disease unless we take into account changes in societal values and social pressures. The definitions of disease found in the 17th and 18th centuries are no longer fully satisfactory in the 20th century.

## III

What constituted the normal or, in the older terminology, the natural? How much variation was allowable? Objective standards evolved slowly, for originally a judgment of something natural rested on personal intuition rather than on measurement. Only in the 19th century did enumeration take a significant part in determining the normal. In large part this determination took place through narrowing the field of reference and specifying the particular character: the normal was defined, say, in respect to bodily temperature, or weight, or cardiac reserve, or bowel function. In determining the normal by enumeration, specifications became more and more narrow and at the same time more and more precise. The establishment of standards could develop through close observation, made easier through measurement and limitation of field.

The concept of normal, however, has several meanings, of which two are especially important in this context. The normal, in the sense of the usual, is determined through enumeration. The other principal meaning involves conformity to type. This represents not an enumeration but a value judgment. It relates to an ideal or to an object of desire.

Substantial deviation from the usual does not of itself indicate disease, as modern statisticians fully realize. Some deviations are highly regarded. Unusual strength is abnormal by definition, but this property could have a high value for society. So, too, with mental endowments. The person who has an intelligence quotient of 180, and the person who can run 100 yards in less than 10 seconds, are both quite outside the normal, but they are not therefore diseased.

On the other hand, a person who has an adult height of only

three feet, or who has six fingers on one hand, is abnormal. The judgment as to whether these divergences indicate disease rests not with the divergence as such but with the decision of society. The grounds for calling a condition a disease rests, ultimately, on the values of society and not on statistical estimation. As we shall see, there are many determining factors that influence such judgments.

The patient with pneumonia or a stroke is obviously diseased, and in these cases pursuing subtle meanings is fruitless. The dwarf or the man with supernumerary digits may or may not be regarded as diseased. Between unmistakable instances of disease and cases of unquestioned health there may be a broad gray zone. This uncertainty, however, arises largely from an ambiguity of language.

In the 16th and 17th centuries, when physicians wrote largely in Latin, they used the word *morbus*, which is translated into English as disease. *Morbus*, however, derives from the Latin *mors*, death. The original sense of *morbus* pointed to a state that might lead to death. This derivation is one reason why the older physicians tended not to include relatively minor states.

The English word "disease" derives from the Old French *aise*, meaning comfort. Dis-ease meant literally the interference with a state of comfort, which is not the same as a serious condition that could lead to death. The difference between *mors* and *aise* accounts for some of the problems of definition. The difficulties arise not from those states which are life-threatening but from those which are unpleasant and yet do not interfere seriously with normal functioning.

The resolution of the problem demands a separation of meanings. We must distinguish two meanings of disease. The one derives from *mors* and threatens death; the other, *dis-ease*, does not relate to death but may interfere with comfort or ease. In the 18th century Hoffmann paid little heed to dis-ease, but, as later authors adopted a more diffuse attitude, the concept of disease merged with the concept of death-threatening ailments.

Societal values play an especial role in identifying states of disease. I will discriminate two types of deviations from health—the serious disease (with no hyphen) and the less serious or even trivial, which I will designate dis-ease. No rigid separation is possible, for there are ramifications and distortions that we must take into account, but a distinction will help to clarify a difficult subject.

There is a continuum between states of dis-ease and states of disease. We can, for example, point to insect bites. The mosquito, in its bite, injects into the skin a substance that produces a complex reaction, one carefully studied by immunologists, biochemists, and physiologists. (I leave out of account, in this discussion, the possible incidental transmission of malaria, yellow fever, or comparable diseases.) A mosquito bite is annoying, it disturbs the peace and contentment of the individual, but we would not ordinarily call the uncomplicated mosquito bite a disease.

Regard now the sting of a bee, which has quite different properties from the material introduced by the mosquito. The bee sting produces in the skin and subcutaneous tissues a complex reaction that also has been much studied. Some persons react only mildly, others intensely. In those who are peculiarly hypersensitive a single sting may cause a fatal anaphylactic reaction. And, even without such idiosyncrasy, multiple stings may produce alarming symptoms and even death.

In most persons a bee sting produces a greater degree of disease than does a mosquito bite, and is more likely to have serious consequences. If, for example, the sting produces a reaction for which a physician needs to administer epinephrine, or antihistamines, or even hydrocortisone, there would, I believe, be general agreement that the victim had a disease. Where will we make the distinction between the mosquito bite and the severe reaction to the bee sting?

We can draw a parallel with sunburn and suntan. Exposure to the sun produces in the skin a complex series of changes whose end result is ordinarily the increase in pigment that we call a tan. This end stage is often considered socially desirable. However, substantial exposure to the sun, even with a selective screening of the sun's rays, is hazardous. Dermatologists warn against excessive exposure to the sun's rays that, in late stages, may produce severe degenerative changes. And in some susceptible persons sunlight induces skin cancer. At the beaches and parks, around swimming pools, on cruise ships, in back yards, we see modern sun worshippers systematically trying to acquire the skin tan they regard as especially pleasing. Many of these sun worshippers, pursuing the desired mahogany hue, produce in their skin severe destructive changes that may not become manifest for twenty years.

Here we have a continuum of changes, some of which are considered socially desirable, while others can fall into the category of disease. Where is the dividing line? How much role does social pressure exert in identifying bodily reactions as disease?

Let us change the scene to advertising on television. Many commercials have to do with pain and discomfort in various modalities: muscular aches, "minor pains of arthritis," headache, "the first sign of a cold," constipation, heartburn, insomnia, "bad breath," to name a few of the most prominent. Some of these may be trivial, others, symptoms of more serious conditions. The advertisements are careful not to make diagnoses. In essence they are encouraging people to be introspective, to note their sensations of discomfort, and then do something about it, namely, buy the recommended product. Implicit is the message: "There is a pill for every ill. You hunt for the ill; we have the pill."

The mere existence of a complaint, trivial or serious, might be considered a prima facie falling-away-from-health. We can accept the concept that by definition any falling-away-from-health is a dis-ease, but that is not the same as disease-as-a-specific-entity, like, say, pneumonia. When we have before us the unqualified term "disease" we must be sure what it refers to, whether to dis-ease, i.e., any-deviation-from-health, trivial or not; or to disease-as-a-specific-entity. The latter we ordinarily qualify by the indefinite or definite article, and we speak of having *a* disease. This concept of entity we will discuss in the next chapter.

IV

Health, for the earlier physicians, meant the ability to perform "natural functions," making due allowance for temperament, age, and sex. The inability to perform these functions indicated disease. Many writers paid no attention to pain as a sign of disease, for certain functions are normally accompanied by pain. We can, for example, point to numerous states of infancy or early childhood. Teething, so far as we can tell, is often painful. Or, when a baby is learning to walk, he falls frequently and falls may be painful. Under such circumstances pain or discomfort are natural, and their presence does not mark any deviation from health.

Childbirth is a function obviously both natural and painful. An intrinsic connection between the two had Biblical warrant: asserted in Genesis, it remained unchallenged in Western thought until the 19th century. The birth process, although painful, was not regarded as a disease. (I am leaving out of account those obstetrical abnormalities always recognized as *contra naturam*.)

The discovery of anaesthesia gave physicians a means of alleviating the pain, but the adoption of anaesthesia had a checkered course. In some circles, especially among men, alleviating the pain of labor was deemed morally wrong and contrary to scripture. The changes in attitude, wherein Queen Victoria played a large part, illustrates the role of social pressure.

In recent times there has been a growing movement to diminish or even eliminate the use of anaesthesia in favor of so-called natural childbirth. The acceptance of considerable pain as normal and even desirable, and the view that natural childbirth, with its attendant discomfort, is preferable to anaesthesia, represents a cultural phenomenon that is itself highly complex. It reflects various social forces that relate to pain, natural function, and disease.

As an added complexity I would point to a recent socio-economic phenomenon. In some instances, employed women who are pregnant may, during their lying-in, receive disability pay, just as for a disabling disease. Are they receiving "sick pay"?

The answer lies with social values, not with medical pronouncements. An affirmative answer does not convert pregnancy into
a disease, but it does show the influence of social pressures on
problems of health. Social values have always played a considerable role in forming the attitudes toward women and the birth
process.

As the last set of examples, I will note certain problems related to personal appearance. These factors are amenable to statistical study. We can gather data on height, weight, and complexion; the size and shape of the nose, of the ears, of the chin;
the alignment of the teeth; the amount and distribution of body
hair; the size and shape of the breasts; the number, type, and
distribution of pigmented spots (as well as areas of depigmen-
tation). All these can be correlated with age, sex, and race. With
the statistics we can easily determine the various ranges and the
deviations therefrom and we can provide distribution curves.
We can determine the influences of both genetic and environmental factors. And, when we are quite finished, we have not
said a word about disease or health.

Personal appearance can cause a great deal of dissatisfaction,
a form of dis-ease. This is particularly the case in relation to
mating behavior. At one time a buxom girl has been considered
especially attractive; at another, the one with a pencil-thin figure. One girl does not like the shape of her nose, another the
bushiness of her eyebrows, another the prominence of her front
teeth. No one would call these conditions a deviation from
health but rather as deviations from the ideals dictated by the
cultural environment of that place and time.

The young man who shows an early onset of male-type baldness, or whose hair turns gray earlier than the average, might,
under certain circumstances, have a disadvantage in coping with
the environment—for example, in finding a suitable job, or
finding a mate, or enjoying ordinary social communion. But to
regard early baldness or premature grayness as disease is running counter to usage and substituting an arbitrary and idiosyn-
cratic viewpoint.

Variations on the normal will, however, show a continuum,

and extreme cases may be considered disease. Facial hirsutism in the female could be such an instance. If resistant to simple cosmetic measures, should the condition be regarded as a disease, and, if so, at what point? Another example would relate to the teeth, with varying degrees of malalignment or malocclusion. At what point would the person be regarded as having a disease? An obvious answer would be when the condition interferes with normal function. But this is exactly the elusive point. Social pressures and the desire to conform to an idealized type are more influential factors than are the physical criteria.

The scientist who studies such conditions and regards them as problems in human biology would correlate the cosmetic appearance with other changes in the body. He studies cellular changes, embryonic development, physico-chemical factors, environmental agents, and genetic determinants. When he has achieved a satisfying correlation, he says he has explained the condition. The explanation renders intelligible the variations in intensity. At no point, however, does he offer a judgment that somewhere along the continuum the condition will be called a disease. Yet such judgments are made. The point on the line where the designation changes is determined by the prevailing culture.

We can also point to a continuum of judgment. Some conditions are universally regarded as disease, as states that lead to death or disability. Disability, however, is not an absolute term. Somewhere there is a distinction between significant and trivial. This distinction, wherever it lies, will depend on the prevailing culture and will vary according to time, place, and cultural patterns.

## CHAPTER 7

# The Clinical Entity and the Disease Entity

*Two people are looking idly at the sky*, watching the clouds. One says, "I see a castle, with a tower, and over there I can see a horse with a man astride, and I can just make out a helmet and a plume." And as he watches, the wind freshens, and he says sadly, "The man has disappeared and the horse has turned into a hill, and the tower of the castle has collapsed." He was drawing on his imagination, forming casual associations with evanescent shapes.

The second man, looking at the sky, says, "This is a typical cumulonimbus cloud, and way over there there is an altostratus cloud." He was not drawing on his imagination. He was naming recurrent well-defined patterns, with specific characteristics. The various properties allow him to identify a given type and discriminate it from others. This man is a meteorologist. He tells his friend the features that distinguish the different formations. The next day the first man, who has learned to identify a few clouds by name, surprises another friend by pointing to the sky and saying, "That is a fine altostratus cloud." The friend, not impressed, says, "So what?" But he received no answer.

The meteorologist, however, can not only identify and name the different kinds of clouds, but he can also tell you a great deal about each one—how it forms and under what circumstances, how it relates to temperature and air currents and moisture content at different levels of the atmosphere. He can tell you what the different formations may indicate about the weather to come. He can tell you about the processes taking place in the atmosphere, both nearby and at a distance. If, after having named a variety of cloud, he were asked, "So what?" he could give a long detailed answer about the *meaning* of that particular cloud and the way it fitted in with other events.

I must emphasize the different aspects of cloud study. On the one hand, we have the process of recognition, identification, and naming. This is really the process of diagnosis that we have considered earlier, wherein the cloud is recognized as belonging to a category with definable properties. The second aspect I call knowledge-about, representing an aggregate of information about that particular class, and constituting its meaning. The two aspects are quite separable. With a little instruction we can learn to recognize several of the chief patterns and to call them by name, but we may be quite ignorant of what they mean. We would not be able to answer that devastating question, "So what?" On the other hand, we might get a book on meteorology and, through reading, learn quite a lot *about* the clouds and the various physical and chemical factors involved; and yet, even with all this knowledge in our heads, we might not be able to make an identification when we look at the sky. Book-learning (for the most part, knowledge-about appears in books) does not necessarily convey skill in identification. Identifying and naming is one process, having information about the entities in question is rather different.

Let us apply this distinction to disease. A physician and a layman friend are in the subway, idly watching the faces of the passengers. In the crowd the physician notes on one man a seborrheic keratosis, on another a basal cell carcinoma. The layman merely notes some lumps that might call up some trivial association, but he could not offer a name. Then they both see a man with a broad vivid red area covering part of his face but stopping sharply at the midline. The layman says, "Oh, that is a port-wine mark." "Yes," says his physician friend, "it is a congenital cutaneous hemangioma." The layman has now learned the technical name for the popular term, port-wine mark. He can make a diagnosis the next time he sees the condition. But, although he can recognize and name, he has no knowledge about the lesion.

If the layman decided to find out all he could about it, he

would learn about cells and tissues and embryology, and the different forces that govern differentiation and the ways that the processes can go wrong. The deeper he got, the more complex the information became and the more the various factors seemed to interdigitate with other branches of knowledge. And, as he faced the enormous mass of accumulated knowledge, he might say to himself, "This is really more than I want to know." And then he might settle for a single textbook of dermatology that describes the condition and gives some relevant information, all in the compass of less than two pages.

"Ah-ha," says the layman, "this gives me a useful core of information about congenital hemangioma, enough to provide a useful understanding when I see the lesion again. Enormous amounts of additional information are available, if I want, that comprise the periphery of the knowledge-about, but for my purposes I can ignore it." His "purpose" did not involve anything more than the satisfaction of curiosity.

In separating recognition from knowledge-about, we might draw a comparison with knowing a person. We can learn to recognize a person, say, an actor, even though his appearance will vary in different situations. There would be a constancy, a basic similarity, so that we get a flash of recognition even in an unfamiliar setting. We imply this in the familiar expression, "Yes, I would recognize him anywhere." So it is with many diseases, which may assume different forms. No two cases are identical, but an experienced physician learns to recognize the condition, even though it is partly concealed in a strange context.

While we may be able to recognize an individual at sight, despite disguises, we do not necessarily know anything about him—his background, his family, his education, his character. These would comprise knowledge about the person, knowledge clearly separable from familiarity with his features or mannerisms. The amount of information about, say, an actor, usually emerges slowly, as biographers dig out and evaluate details. We call this research. Once the biographer starts digging, the ramifications and interconnections know no limits.

I labor this point because of its extreme importance in under-standing the terms "clinical entity" and "disease entity" that play such an important part in medical theory.

When the layman spoke of a port-wine mark and then learned to substitute the technical term "congenital cutaneous heman-gioma," he was pointing to a clinical entity. In this chapter I mean by the word "entity" only something that serves as a sub-ject of discourse, that we can talk about in a meaningful fashion. We must not confuse "entity" with "thing." The latter has the connotation of a material object, but three-dimensional materi-ality is not at all of the essence. An idea, a concept, a relation-ship, all purely immaterial, may also be designated as entities just as much as a spleen or a bacterium. For our present pur-poses, an entity may be a recurrent pattern, a unique historical event, a three-dimensional object; it may be conceptual or ma-terial, past or present. But, in any case, we can talk about it in a meaningful way.

The term "clinical" is somewhat simpler. The word derives from the Greek *klinē*, meaning bed. The original context re-ferred to a patient sick enough to stay in bed and to be seen by a physician, who was a *klinikos*. Clinical referred to medical practice at the bedside. We can think of the vanished days when the patient, sick at home, would call the physician, who would then come to the house, make his observations, and direct treat-ment, all at the bedside. By extension the term also applied to the ambulatory patient who might visit the doctor's office rather than having the doctor visit him. In either case the essential meaning had to do with the direct relationship between the pa-tient and his physician.

The clinical entity permits a contrast with disease entity. I suggest the following tentative distinction. The clinical entity is a recurrent pattern having to do with disease; it is a gestalt or configuration that stands out as a unit and can be recognized as a unit. The emphasis lies with the concepts of pattern and of recognition. By implication there is a special association with the doctor-patient relationship, with the physician trying to *do* something for the patient. The concept has to do essentially with the practice of medicine.

The disease entity, on the other hand, is the clinical entity with a large accretion of knowledge-about. Such knowledge helps us to understand the condition, how it came into being, how it relates to various other factors, various other states. As knowledge-about accumulates, it may prove valuable in the care of the patient and force us to modify the original concept of the clinical entity. How much knowledge-about we must have to justify the term disease entity is a moot point.

Whence arises the knowledge-about? One principal source was direct observation at the bedside. The physician, who might see many patients with the same ailment, could compare, note similarities and differences, and make generalizations. We see this process, for example, in the *Aphorisms* of Hippocrates. There were also post-mortem examinations, whereby the state of the internal organs could be correlated with the bedside findings and the course of the disease. Such correlations stimulated explanatory hypotheses and theories of causation.

Another source was the study, not directly of the patient but rather of the attendant circumstances and environmental factors. The simplest example concerns malaria, which even two thousand five hundred years ago was recognized as an unmistakable clinical entity. Observers noted a peculiar relation to the environment, namely, an especial prevalence in the vicinity of marshes and swamps and an increased incidence in the summer months.

Other sources of knowledge included laboratory studies. Although we ordinarily think of the laboratory as a modern institution, the ancient Greeks made observations that must be recognized as laboratory data. The criterion, I believe, would be the *indirect* examination of the patient, wherein the physician attended not immediately to the patient but to some separable aspect of the patient, such as his urine or feces or vomitus. Hippocrates recommended these observations, especially the study of the urine.

From examination of the urine Hippocrates reached conclusions expressed as aphorisms: "Blood or pus in the urine indicates ulceration of the kidneys or of the bladder. . . . Thick urine containing bran-like particles indicates inflammation of the bladder. . . . A sandy urinary sediment shows that a stone is forming in the bladder."[1]

Knowledge increased greatly through progress in the basic medical sciences that expanded especially in the 17th century and have progressed in geometrical ratio ever since. Much of this progress derived from experimental studies, whether on animals or in vitro. Increased knowledge of anatomy, physiology, chemistry, and pathology enlarged the understanding of disease conditions. Today more and more of our knowledge-about comes from deliberate experiments, whose interpretations depend on theory engendered by earlier experiments and observations.

A textbook of medicine provides us with a survey of disease entities. In discussing various diseases it will present for each the knowledge-about that happens to be considered important at the time: the mechanisms by which the disease arises (often known as the pathogenesis), the theories of causation, the various factors that exert an influence, the relationships to comparable conditions, the means of making a diagnosis. These accounts vary in length. One book will present a subject in a page, another in ten or fifteen pages. Then there are whole books dealing with a single disease.

All this is knowledge-about, but the quantity presented will depend on the audience for whom the book is designed. The paramedical personnel, the medical student, the practicing physician, the specialist, the research worker, will all want different amounts of knowledge-about. Different aspects of the total will have different degrees of relevance, according to the particular purpose in view. What is suitable for one will be excessive—or perhaps insufficient—for another.

Knowledge-about, providing information that aids in understanding, necessarily involves theory. And theories change. An excellent way to appreciate medical history is to study the way that successive authors expound a given disease entity. Chapter

2, above, a brief review of a single disease, permits us to appreciate the progressive changes in our knowledge-about. We have no reason to doubt that our present-day explanations will undergo comparable change, so that the future will hold a different view of the disease entity.

With all the changes in theory, the clinical entity remains relatively constant (at least, in some instances). Hippocrates described the clinical entity puerperal fever in terms so precise, so vivid, that even twenty-five hundred years later we have no difficulty in reaching a diagnosis from the data he presented. Thomas Sydenham, in the 17th century, gave us a magnificent description of clinical gout that can scarcely be improved on today. There are many "classic descriptions of disease." The crucial word here is "description." That which is described is relatively constant. The variable is the explanation offered.

In an important paper published in 1949, Otto Guttentag offers insights into these concepts. The clinical entity relates to those factors which a physician observes. It is patient-oriented, "a concept that has been created and is perpetuated by physicians to facilitate diagnostic and therapeutic approaches to the individual patient. . . . The actual sets of phenomena that constitute such an arrangement [i.e., pattern, in my terminology] vary at different historical periods."[2]

There have always been theories to explain the pattern, and these theories, I suggest, have to do with the science of medicine. The theories change through the ages. "It is the clinical entity which bridges the gap between these different theories . . . it is relatively far removed from the background of theoretical speculation." The clinical entity would thus be a persistent thread among the shifting theories.

I would emphasize, however, that a distinction between the practice of medicine and the theories of medicine is approximate and not absolute, and so too with the distinction between the clinical entity and the disease entity. I would phrase the difference in this fashion: the clinical entity is the category through which we identify a discrete pattern of illness, while the disease entity is the category by which we understand the illness. To make an identification we may need only a few data or we may need a lot, but there is always patient-orientation. For the disease entity the data may extend quite without limit, but will show varying degrees of relevance. Greater understanding then enables us to make discriminations within a clinical entity.

## II

Which conditions should we call clinical entities and which ones disease entities? When should we consider two or more clinically distinguishable states to be a single disease? Our answers relate to our attitudes toward the basic nature of medicine.

Let us examine some concrete instances. In Chapter 2 I discussed both consumption (or phthisis) and scrofula. These are quite distinct clinical entities. They attack different age groups, show a different clinical course, prognosis, and pathological manifestations. Yet they also show certain relationships, clinically and pathologically. Physicians had long disputed whether they were two disease entities or might be construed as variations on a single theme.

The discovery of the tubercle bacillus did not really solve the problem. Further research soon identified different kinds of tubercle bacilli. The type that ordinarily infected cattle (*Mycobacterium bovis*) could also infect man, usually through the alimentary tract. Then it produced the clinical picture known as scrofula. When tuberculosis in cattle was virtually eliminated, the clinical entity scrofula almost vanished.

Phthisis, the form of pulmonary tuberculosis formerly called consumption, resulted from infection with a different species of bacteria, namely, *M. tuberculosis*, whose portal of entry was usually the respiratory tract. *M. bovis* and *M. tuberculosis* are quite distinguishable, but they are also closely related. Hence it occasions no surprise that in man the two clinical pictures, usually distinct, might show considerable overlap.

How, then, should we answer the question: "Are scrofula and phthisis, clinically distinct, two separate disease entities?" The answer depends on the context of inquiry. The epidemiologist and the worker in public health will consider scrofula quite

distinct from pulmonary tuberculosis. The internist will probably regard them as variants of the same disease, and the lecturer
who teaches second-year medical students will almost certainly
stress the similarity. We can answer "yes" or "no" as the context
demands. This context relates to the purpose for which the discrimination is made and the usefulness of the answer in achieving that purpose. In any definition of the disease entity, the
concepts of usefulness and purpose are crucial.

A somewhat comparable example we find in malaria, well
recognized in ancient times. Hippocrates distinguished certain
clinical types—the quotidian, the tertian, and the quartan, depending on the periodicity of the paroxysms. The discovery of
the specific infectious agent, the plasmodium, opened the door
to a clearer understanding, and permitted sharper clinical differentiation. The distinguishable clinical patterns were fairly
well correlated with three distinct species of plasmodium. Bor-
derline and atypical cases continued to complicate the picture,
but to a much less degree than formerly. Occasionally, the laboratory could identify in man an unusual species of plasmodium
that did not, however, show a distinctive clinical course. These
unusual species could not be correlated with any distinctive clinical entity, as could the major types. The manifestations tended
to merge with the other types, and only the laboratory could
indicate the unusual nature of the infecting agent.

In what we call malaria, how many entities do we want to
distinguish? Should we consider each of the three main clinical
types a separate disease entity? Should an unusual species, with
no distinct clinical pattern, also be considered a disease entity?
For ordinary medical practice this would be unbearable pedantry; for certain investigative purposes it might not be.

A very different example, and in a sense the converse of malaria, would be "food poisoning," long a well-recognized clinical entity. Progress in bacteriology had shown that this could
result from a variety of infectious agents. A great range of different bacteria can induce diarrhea, fever, prostration, and related symptoms. While an experienced clinician might make a
reasonable guess regarding the major class of responsible bac-

teria, his opinion would remain little more than a guess. Only the laboratory could offer precision.

Among the bacteria that cause gastroenteritis is the genus *Salmonella*. Scientists in the laboratory can clearly distinguish hundreds of different types or species, but there is no way to make a comparable clinical distinction. A fairly uniform clinical picture may result from hundreds of distinguishable bacterial agents. Will each separate species of *Salmonella* represent a separate disease entity comparable to *M. bovis* and *M. tuberculosis?* At present this would be meaningless pedantry, serving no discernible purpose.

A still different example we find in puerperal fever, which, as we have already noted, was well recognized by Hippocrates. Today we speak of a diffuse peritonitis usually due to a streptococcus, while less frequently some other organism is involved. We can now distinguish a diffuse infection of the peritoneum from a more localized infection, and distinguish further a bacterial infection from an aseptic febrile reaction that might arise, say, from a retention of lochia.

These important clinical distinctions that an obstetrician makes today were not possible in an earlier era. Instead, different conditions were lumped together as variations in the diffuse entity, childbed fever. Discrimination became possible only when bacteriology, anatomy, pathology, and physiology enriched and, so to speak, fertilized the earlier clinical observations. The enrichment permitted physicians to discriminate entities that previously had been fused together.

Should we call childbed fever a disease entity? This problem severely worried Philippe Pinel (1755-1826), who knew nothing whatever of bacteria, but was concerned with the question of classification. He refused to grant childbed fever the status of a separate disease, but regarded it as merely the focus of other factors that included the true disease. He presented an interesting argument: during pregnancy and the puerperium women are in a special physiological state that renders them peculiarly susceptible. "Pregnancy and lying-in alter the constitution of the woman so as to make her liable to all the diseases epidemic in

the environment where she happens to be. The onset of dentition, the first menstruation, the no less formidable period of the
menopause, bring about remarkable changes in the organism,
and render the child and the woman susceptible to most diseases,
and are also responsible for their greater intensity."[3]

According to Pinel, what we today would call physiological
stress renders a woman susceptible to whatever diseases are prevalent at the time. There was no more reason, he thought, for
regarding puerperal fever as a separate entity than there would
be to identify a fever of dentition, a pubertal fever, a menopau-
sal fever, or a fever of breast feeding. Puerperal fever is nothing more than the name for the innumerable febrile diseases that
attack the newly delivered woman. Pregnancy and lying-in
would thus be a predisposing factor for any sort of fever.

Today, with our vastly increased knowledge, we still face the
same problem that Pinel faced. Is puerperal fever a disease entity? Or should we say that the disease entity is the streptococcus
infection that happened to localize in the female genital tract and
then spread to the peritoneum? Then we note that erisypelas, a
distinct clinical entity, is also a streptococcus infection. Even
when we make allowances for the differences in bacterial type,
should we regard erisypelas and puerperal fever as the same
disease entity? We may lump them together if we want, or we
may keep them distinct, depending on the purpose that we have
in mind. Defining the disease entity is an arbitrary process dependent on context, interest, and usefulness.


### III

So far the examples have been drawn from infectious diseases,
a category that makes relatively easy any discussion of the disease
entity. Infections are all characterized by some concrete transmissible agent, often called the "cause," which, according to
some views, provides fixity and stability. We find a much
greater difficulty in analyzing the non-infectious diseases, wherein,
it so happens, the "cause" refuses to be pinned down. As a
result, the non-infectious diseases are especially important for

understanding the disease entity. I will present briefly three examples to illustrate some of the major difficulties.

A condition often called heart-block was fairly well defined in the early 19th century. It is ordinarily associated with the names of Robert Adams (1781-1875) and William Stokes (1804-1878), who offered brief descriptions in 1827 and 1846, respectively. The striking clinical features were the loss of consciousness, often with convulsions, associated with a very slow pulse. The early reports, purely clinical and descriptive, offered no explanatory data, and hence, in the framework of the present discussion, would designate a clinical entity. Writers who have no objection to eponyms often speak of Adams-Stokes disease (or sometimes of Adams-Stokes syndrome). Writers who dislike eponyms prefer the terminology "complete heart-block."

A condition with such striking clinical features attracted a great deal of attention. Investigation of the relevant anatomy and pathology soon yielded a great deal of knowledge-about, which could explain the clinical findings. The normal heart rhythm is established in a special mass of tissue in the right atrium. Special bands of conducting tissue transfer the impulses from the atrium to the ventricles. If the conduction bundle is interrupted, the normal cardiac rhythm is not transmitted to the ventricles, which then exhibit a much slower autonomous beat. The total output of blood into the arteries is thereby diminished. Inadequate output may lead to inadequate blood supply for the brain, and this in turn reveals itself in various signs, ranging from weakness and loss of consciousness to convulsions. The clinician readily detects the slowed heart rate by feeling the pulse.

Our modern knowledge was not available to Adams or Stokes. They described a pure clinical entity that has since become extremely well explained. Heart-block is unequivocally both a clinical entity and a disease entity, sharply defined, clearly recognized, and well explained through a coherent body of relevant scientific data.

If we demand "etiology" in order to define a disease entity, and if we ask, "What *causes* heart block?" we would answer,

"The interruption of the conduction bundles." And if we further ask, "What causes this interruption?" then the clarity oozes away. There might be destruction of the specialized bundles, with replacement by scar tissue. This might in turn result from arteriosclerosis or it might follow some inflammatory reaction in the heart (a true myocarditis). And these, in their turn, might have many inciting factors. Shall we therefore say that the disease entity is "really" arteriosclerosis (or perhaps an infection, or an allergic inflammation)? Such queries lead to confusion.

Much of this confusion arises from the mistaken belief that we can classify our diseases on the basis of cause. The futility of such an expectation was fully recognized in the 18th century, but our great scientific progress in the interim has masked that futility. The problem I will discuss in detail in the analysis of causation.

My second example is Graves' disease, an early name for a condition now included under hyperthyroidism. Robert Graves (1797-1853) described it in 1835, while C. A. von Basedow (1789-1854) also noted many features in 1840. Historians associate other names with the early delineation of the entity. Graves clearly indicated some of the salient points: enlargement of the thyroid gland, rapid heart rate, sweating and other "nervous" complaints, pretibial edema, and other manifestations of which protrusion of the eyeballs was the most prominent.

The early writers described a coherent pattern of symptoms but without any explanation. The understanding of the condition lagged until the 20th century, when endocrinology developed as a discipline in its own right. At present, immunology and physiological chemistry have taken center stage in clarifying the entity that Graves and others had described.

While the original term "exophthalmic goitre" has a descriptive value, the condition has since become embedded in a larger whole, "hyperthyroidism" or "thyrotoxicosis." Excessive thyroid function shows a spectrum of manifestations, and Graves' disease, as originally described, directs attention to only a portion of that total range. Through highly specialized technology modern medicine can determine many types and degrees of hyperthyroidism and many clinically separable ways in which it may become manifest. Clinicians recognize, among other states, the diffuse hyperplastic goitre, the solitary hyperplastic nodule, and the toxic multi-nodular goitre. Are they all manifestations of a single underlying disease state, or should we regard them as discrete entities? They have features in common but also significant features in which they differ.

As originally described, Adams-Stokes disease and Graves' disease both refer to clinical patterns, but the former has remained quite stable, as new knowledge developed. Physicians noted lesser degrees of heart-block, called incomplete heart-block, that did not show the full clinical entity that Adams and Stokes described. Yet, even with the expansion of cases and the wealth of explanatory data that has accrued, the original entity could accommodate the new information without strain. The original pattern enlarged but did so without much distortion.

The original pattern that Graves described also expanded as physicians recognized new varieties of hyperthyroidism. But, as the original concept expanded and we learned more and more about the mechanisms involved, the pattern showed signs of strain. The broader concept of hyperthyroidism makes us recognize the limitations of the original description.

As a third example I offer a pattern that proved to be extremely unstable, namely Bright's disease. Richard Bright (1789-1858) called attention to three manifestations that seemed to hang together as a feature of kidney disease. He pointed to dropsy, albumin in the urine, and structural changes in the kidney. These, he indicated, had an inner coherence. Each of these components, in isolation, had been familiar to physicians. It was Bright's great contribution to perceive the connection among the three and to point out that they formed a recurrent pattern with an inner togetherness. Bright's disease quickly became an accepted term in the French and German literature, as well as in the English.

Bright's disease was not strictly a clinical entity, for it included pathological observations that at that time could be noted only at autopsy. He combined clinical and pathological observations, welding them into an entity that proved rather unstable. Within his original descriptions we can now perceive several distinct sub-groups, each with its own characteristics. The original pattern began to fragment into subordinate patterns, including varieties of glomerulonephritis, nephrosis, and types of shrunken kidneys having quite different origins.

Pathologists, physiologists, and biochemists, working intensively, made enormous progress in understanding the structure and function of the kidneys under different conditions. However, the various scientific data did not correlate too well with clinical features. Numerous subordinate patterns were proposed, but without general agreement. Indeed, in the history of medicine the classification of kidney diseases has been an extremely thorny subject. What Bright assumed to be a unit turned out to be highly composite, and his original entity, useful within a limited context, soon lost its value.

We can compare Bright's disease with the consumption of the 17th century. Morton had circumscribed a recognizable pattern and indicated criteria for its identification. But the pattern as originally propounded applied equally well to several other entities, such as cancer and lung abscess, that later became sharply distinguished. Morton's concept proved useful for a limited period until the growth of knowledge showed the need for more precise discrimination. So too with Bright's concept. The pattern he described proved useful and valid for a limited period, but as a result of medical progress gave way to other more distinct entities. Unlike Adams-Stokes disease, Bright's original pattern could not accommodate itself to increased knowledge.

## IV

The clinical entity, a pattern of symptoms, becomes a disease entity when enough information has accumulated to explain the pattern. Explanation ordinarily involves theoretical elaboration that provides a sense of order and understanding, that relates, for example, the observed symptoms to the data resulting from scientific investigation.[4] The disease entity is thus a construct that renders experience orderly.

Disease entities are the units that make up a textbook of medicine, and correspondingly the units of classification. This was entirely obvious in an earlier period, when nosology was a more popular term. The nosologies classified disease entities as they were then understood. However, discrimination between clinical and disease entities is relatively modern, for it reflects especially the enormous increase in knowledge-about, resulting from the expansion of scientific studies.

As knowledge changes, what has been accepted at one time may no longer find acceptance. Since the disease entity, as a concept, renders limited areas of experience orderly and intelligible, it enables us to handle it in a satisfactory manner. But what we call a disease entity has variable degrees of stability, and as knowledge expands the older concepts may no longer permit a satisfactory handling of experience. Then physicians and scientists devise a new concept. This has been abundantly illustrated in Chapter 2. The original entity may break up into two or more. In other conditions perhaps two or more concepts, once considered distinct, may get fused into a more comprehensive unity. Or a new pattern may be perceived, as occurred when the concept of the ultra-microscopic virus finally entered into bacteriological thought.

At this point I would mention the distinction between a symptom and a disease. Any acquaintance with the history of medicine brings to mind the change in status that has overtaken various concepts. At one time fever was regarded as a disease, and so too with inflammation or jaundice. Now we regard them as symptoms. There need be no confusion. A symptom is a component of some pattern we call a disease. A disease is a pattern in its own right. Jaundice, for example, was at one time considered to be such a pattern, which satisfactorily ordered the medical experience of the day. With additional data and further observation this alleged pattern, instead of making things orderly, led to confusion. Re-establishing the sense of order required a new concept, and the status of jaundice was reduced, from independence to a component of other patterns.

There remains for consideration the term "syndrome," which means literally a running together or a concurrence. The concurrence refers to individual symptoms. The term has become extremely popular in the last half century or so. It presupposes the concept of disease entity, i.e., the distinguishable pattern about which we have some considerable amount of information. As early as 1855 a syndrome was properly regarded as an enumeration of symptoms "without any necessary connection to discrete disease" (*sans rapport obligé à des maladies determinées*).[5]

According to this author every individual case that the practitioner sees need not fit into the framework of recognized diseases as found in a text of medicine. Instances that seem anomalous should be identified, but in a manner less rigid (*determinée*) than in a formal nosological classification. In this view a syndrome would be a category intermediate between a formally defined disease entity that has found a place in a textbook and an unclassified individual case. The term "syndrome" thus provides a tentative mode of identification. It refers to an ailment that attracts attention through some unusual combination of symptoms but does not match any well-recognized disease entity. A physician creates a syndrome when he asserts that a cluster of phenomena, instead of being a random aggregate, has some inner connection that indicates a unity. The physician thereby asserts a pattern and removes the case from the domain of the random to the domain of the orderly.

In a syndrome there may be little or even negligible knowledge-about. When such knowledge-about does accumulate, the syndrome may or may not receive the designation of disease. The transitional point is entirely indefinite and depends on circumstances. I would, however, strongly reject any assertion or implication that a syndrome is a condition for which "the cause" has not yet been found, or that a syndrome "becomes" a disease when "the cause" is found. This is totally repugnant to historical usage, and involves confusion regarding causation, especially between "a cause" and "the cause."

For reasons that may be venal, recent years have witnessed a tremendous pressure to identify and publish new syndromes. Hundreds, probably thousands, have been identified. However, syndrome and clinical entity merge imperceptibly with each other. When an undetermined amount of relevant knowledge-about accumulates, the syndrome or the clinical entity assumes a position as a disease entity. The syndrome and the clinical entity are useful in identifying patterns, the disease entity in understanding them. All three terms serve a useful function. Whenever they lose their usefulness, whenever that function can be better served by some different pattern or concept, then the entity will change, perhaps disappear, or get transformed in one or another way.

Medical terminology is a language, constantly growing and changing, and language does not tolerate a straitjacket. We can compare syndromes, clinical entities, and disease entities to words in a dictionary. Some words, with venerable continuity, have a rich meaning, with many shadings accumulated over the years. Some of these shadings are listed as obsolete. A syndrome would be comparable to a new word, coined in response to a new-felt need, but with a sharply limited meaning. If new words gain general acceptance, they will in time expand their meaning. Words not accepted will become obsolete.

Medical concepts cease to be current when they cease to perform a useful function. We cannot regard them as rigid entities to be shut up in little boxes that then may be stacked, labelled, and classified. Labels are indeed a practical necessity, and so are classifications, but the concepts they represent are constantly changing, even if imperceptibly.

Many physicians find this brute fact abhorrent and they try to achieve a standard nomenclature so that the terms may be stable and uniform. For many purposes this is highly desirable. Such compendia can serve specific practical requirements, such as hospital record-keeping, or vital statistics, or filling out insurance forms. The various standard codifications are useful within the practical context for which they were designed. But we must appreciate the limitations. If a classification, designed for a definite purpose, gets applied to some other area for which it was not designed, the result may be disastrous.

Meaning is relative to use, and for *specific practical purposes* we can ignore the essential fluidity. But to understand the nature of disease we cannot ignore the fluidity; we must not be misled by artificial classifications that, instead of promoting overall comprehension, may slowly strangle the understanding.

CHAPTER 8

When, Where, and What Is the Disease?

I

*When Is the Disease?*

Until about a half century ago the term "crisis" was commonly used in medicine. The word itself means a decision, a point of decisive change. At the crisis the patient would either pass the danger point and get well or he would get worse and die. A dramatic example of a crisis often occurred in lobar pneumonia, when the desperately sick patient could take a sudden turn for the better—or else for the worse. Similar turning points are seen in many febrile diseases. The layman might use the expression, "the fever broke"; the pathologist and immunologist can give a complex explanation that depends on antibodies and cellular defenses.

In times past the physicians made much of this decisive and relatively sudden change in the patient's condition. The ancient Greeks, keen observers, noted that episodes of change would often bear a definite time relationship to the onset of the disease. The seventh day and the multiples of seven seemed to have a special significance, and, if the crisis did not occur on the seventh day, it might take place on the fourteenth. Different diseases, however, might show variation in the critical day.[1]

Until relatively recently the physician, in treating infectious diseases, provided chiefly supportive and symptomatic therapy. He could not do much to affect the disease directly. Hence, when the laity tried to evaluate the merits of a physician, an important criterion was his ability to foretell what would happen. If he could predict accurately, his reputation would rise. Accurate forecasting, rather than absolute cure rate, distin-

guished the good physician from the mediocre one. Predicting
the critical day would indicate to the anxious family how much
longer the suspense would last and when the family might learn
that the patient was out of danger. When I was a medical student, this mode of thinking manifested itself by placing the
patient "on the danger list." When the patient had passed the
critical stage, he was removed from the danger list. Today, with
our overflowing technology, we substitute the impressive term
"intensive care."

Knowledge that a crisis would probably occur was one thing;
ability to predict the day on which it would occur was something
else. Critical days were counted from the "beginning" of the
illness. But when did the disease begin? In earlier times this was
not merely an exercise in logic-chopping but a real problem.
The answer could make a real difference to the family as well
as to the reputation of the physician.

Knowing when the disease began could also have practical
importance in therapy. In one of the earliest statistical studies of
disease Pierre Louis (1787-1872) examined the effectiveness of
blood-letting in pneumonia.[2] Prior to his work, phlebotomy was
the prevalent treatment, but used without much discrimination.
Louis, for the first time, did a statistical analysis to seek objective evidence on the subject. He found that the effectiveness of
blood-letting depended on its relation to the onset of the disease.
According to his analysis, phlebotomy had therapeutic value
only if carried out in the first two days of the disease.

Louis' "numerical method," a landmark study, contained
many fallacies that need not concern us now. For our purposes
the relevant feature involves the onset of the disease, to serve as
the base-line for determining the effectiveness of phlebotomy.
With lobar pneumonia a relatively sudden attack of chills, pain
in the chest, and fever marks a dramatic change in condition,
while a sniffling coryza for a few days before or a vague indisposition might easily get overlooked. Even though in some cases
the symptoms might appear more gradually, the severe changes
usually had a sharply demarcated onset. Louis thus had a more
or less uniform point of reference. However, we may distinguish the prominent symptoms from the disease itself and ask,

"When did the *disease* start?" Let us examine some temporal aspects of disease.

Ordinarily in clinical medicine, the precise onset of a disorder we know only in cases of sudden accidents and injuries. Some readers may not want to use the term "disease" to describe an automobile accident or a bullet wound, but I see no objection to this nomenclature, nor any essential difference between the damage done by a sudden violent physical force and the damage done more gradually by an invading bacterium or virus, faulty diet, or hostile environment.

To identify the beginning of a disease the early physicians had to rely exclusively on what they could observe for themselves and what the patients reported. This information was expanded through post-mortem examination, whereby the pathologist could correlate clinical observation and anatomical change and could also make inferences regarding stages prior to the complaint.[3] In tuberculosis, as we have seen, Bayle used post-mortem studies to emphasize the concept of process. He stressed the lesions that might have existed before symptoms were manifest. We call this a sub-clinical stage, i.e., changes that cannot be appreciated at the bedside but are inferred from other data, gathered by other methods. This is one of the most fruitful of all medical concepts: that disease is a continuous process whose beginnings exist prior to clinical manifestations. This concept has helped to mark the difference between the disease entity and the clinical entity.

Experimental studies introduced a new dimension in the understanding of disease and led not only to new information but to new attitudes. When an investigator injects an infectious agent into a susceptible host, he has precise control over the beginning of the disease. He can thus study accurately the reactions induced by the agent and the early bodily changes. The more delicate the techniques, the more he can learn. There has been a continuous progression to more precise techniques—gross pathology, microscopy, ultramicroscopic changes, immunological phenomena, and chemical alterations. And techniques for more exact discriminations are constantly expanding.

As the research worker studies the continuity of disease process, he finds that at some point the symptoms will become apparent to the direct and unaided senses. Suppose, for example, we inject twenty mice with a suspension of a virus, such as equine encephalomyelitis. Immediately thereafter the injected animals are indistinguishable from the controls. But after, say, forty-eight or seventy-two hours, they may appear sluggish; they may sit hunched in a corner, with their fur ruffled. They are obviously "sick." So too with guinea pigs. The inoculated animals may at first be indistinguishable from normal controls, but the rectal temperature may go up sharply when no other change is detectable. The ruffled fur of the mice, the rise in temperature of the guinea pigs, would be *clinical* symptoms of disease.

However, more precise studies would show subtle bodily changes prior to the clinical symptoms. During the incubation period—the interval between the inoculation and the appearance of the first clinical symptoms—specific techniques will show many alterations. The virus had multiplied. It spread from the site of inoculation into the blood and then had been deposited in various organs. The degree and mode of spread would vary with the agent and the host. These findings, however, are discovered not by simple clinical observation but only by experimental means and special techniques. All these findings comprise knowledge about the disease and help to shape our concept of the disease entity.

We would have no hesitation, I believe, in saying that the disease started with the inoculation and progressed first in a subclinical manner, and then with overt and clinically observable symptoms. But the changes that took place in the incubation period are just as much manifestations of the disease process as are the later florid changes that forcefully call attention to themselves and comprise the clinical entity. If, as is historically proper, we regard symptom and manifestation as strictly synonymous, then we say that the changes during the incubation period are symptoms of the disease, but *symptoms that require special techniques for their demonstration.* By definition they are not *clinical* symptoms, but they are symptoms nevertheless.

Let us examine some of the further implications. Suppose that we inoculate twenty animals, and only fifteen of them become obviously and clinically "sick." The remaining five showed no clinical symptoms. Did they "have" the disease? Obviously, clinical acumen alone cannot answer the question. Suppose, however, through delicate techniques for detecting antibodies, we find that three animals, showing no overt symptoms, nevertheless did develop specific antibodies against the injected virus. We would say that the animals had a *latent infection*. The virus had induced a defense reaction in the body, and these defenses could overcome the infecting virus before the unaided senses could detect any change. The concept of a latent infection has enlarged our concept of the disease entity.

Suppose, however, that of the animals showing no overt symptoms, two had no evidence of antibody protection. Available techniques provided no evidence that the injected agent had induced any reaction. We would then have no grounds for asserting that these animals had a latent infection. The evidence, of course, might have been too subtle for our available methods, but within the limits of our knowledge we would say that these two animals did not have the disease.

The experimenter is a scientist who aims to advance knowledge, not to treat a particular patient. His concept of the disease will not coincide with that of the clinician. Fever and malaise are manifestations of disease, but so too is the production of antibodies. Some manifestations are readily observable, others require high technology. Some manifestations are especially relevant to the work of the clinician, others especially relevant to the task of the scientist. The activities of the clinician and the scientist overlap to some extent, and there is no sharp line of division except in the problem of goal or intent.

In clinical medicine, then, except in unusual cases, we are quite unable to answer the question, "When did the disease start?" We can know when the patient started to complain, for he can often tell with considerable accuracy when he first perceived discomfort or became uneasy over a physical finding. But this, of course, only marks a particular point in a process that had already been in existence. For example, if we are dealing with an infection, we assume that the disease began when the patient came in contact with the infectious agent. If a child exposed to another child with mumps becomes sick with mumps two weeks later, we may safely date the beginning of the illness to the time of exposure.

Infectious diseases, however, are only a small part of medical practice. If we think of diabetes, hypertension, coronary arteriosclerosis, gout, or cancer, we have no way of telling when the disease began. We can only know when the patient first became aware of some manifestation, or else when the physician found evidence of which the patient had not been conscious.

Physicians frequently encounter diseases of which the patient had been totally unaware. At an autopsy the pathologist will almost always find traces of some disease that had no clinical counterpart. Most dramatic for the general public is the so-called silent cancer, discovered, ordinarily, by a surgeon, a radiologist, or a pathologist. Such a condition represents a subclinical disease in a state comparable, I suggest, to the incubation period of an infection. The silent cancer is a good example of the disease entity that is not yet a clinical entity.

A somewhat different illustration in temporal relationships would be a woman who, with no complaints at all, is found on routine examination to have an abnormal cervical smear. We can give her condition a name, "cervical dysplasia." This descriptive term indicates an abnormal pattern of the cervical epithelium. Some cases return to normal under simple hygienic treatment, other cases go on to cancer despite such hygienic regime. We cannot say that the woman has cancer. At most we would say that she has a tendency toward cancer, a tendency to which we can assign a probability level based on prior statistical study.

Suppose that the condition remains untreated and does in fact progress to cancer. When did the cancer start? Was it present all the time, concealed by the cover-all diagnosis "dysplasia"? Perhaps the dysplasia was "really" cancer all the time. We have no means of answering these questions. Since we have neither the theoretical knowledge nor the technology for making a discrimination, we are in a position strictly comparable to that of the 18th-century physician making a diagnosis of scirrhus.[4]

Now consider the man who, on routine examination, is found to have a high uric acid level in his blood, but no other findings, subjective or objective, referable to gout. Does he "have" gout? Certainly not in the sense of a clinical entity. If, however, ten years later he shows characteristic symptoms of that disease, can we say that he "had" gout at the time of the first examination? If not, when did the gout begin?

Only rarely can we find a meaningful answer to the question, "When did the disease begin?" I suggest two possible reasons for the inability. Perhaps our technology is not sufficiently precise to identify the moment when the change from normal to abnormal took place. On the other hand, we can properly say that relationships are so intertwined that any attempt at precise demarcation is philosophically unsound, arbitrary, and always dependent on a particular context; any attempt to give a precise answer is a false simplicity, intrinsically wrong, even though often practically useful.

## II

*Where Is the Disease?*

Correlative to the query "When?" is the further question, "*Where* is the disease?" Supposedly, every disease had its own "seat" or site. The great work of Giovanni Battista Morgagni (1682-1781) bore the title, *De Sedibus et Causis Morborum* (1761), translated as *The Seats and Causes of Diseases*. These were "investigated by anatomy," that is, through morphological changes found in the various organs. The book dealt with different loci—the head, the thorax, the abdomen, the extremities—and, within each grouping, discussed the different diseases affecting the one or another part. Some diseases, however, such as "fevers," were considered to affect the whole body. As generalized conditions, they did not have a localized site.[5]

The attempt to find a *place* where the disease was acting encountered difficulties, since any given site had component parts.

Did the disease involve an individual component that we call a tissue, or a cluster of tissues that we call an organ? The ancient anatomists clearly distinguished the organs from the component tissues, although they used a different nomenclature. Under the influence of Galen, physicians had identified "similar parts," such as muscles, bones, nerves, blood vessels, and the like. These had each a homogeneity and served as anatomical elements. These were distinguished from "dissimilar parts," where different elements combined into functional wholes, such as the arm or the face; or into organs like the liver or kidney. What we call organs comprised an aggregate of similar parts (like blood vessels or nerves), together with a characteristic matter unique for each organ, known as the parenchyma of that organ. The old physicians distinguished clearly among diseases. Some would involve the similar parts, others the dissimilar parts, and the relationships had to do with the concept of substantial form that I have discussed at length elsewhere.[6]

In the 17th century the older Galenic ideas receded into the background, and precise studies of anatomy and pathology underwent a tremendous expansion over the next two hundred years. The pathology of whole organs became discriminated into tissue pathology. Xavier Bichat (1771-1802), without benefit of microscopy, founded the science of histology, which clarified the older concepts.

The early pathologists attended only to relatively severe changes. Those organs which did not show substantial gross changes were regarded as normal or, in the language of the 18th century, "natural." With experience, however, pathologists could identify, through gross examination, even quite modest changes from the normal. Then the development of microscopy permitted recognition of subtle changes where gross alterations were not perceptible.

In the 19th century, anatomical pathology, both gross and microscopic, provided the principal data to correlate with the clinical findings and to explain the clinical entity. However, physiology and chemistry gradually contributed more and more to clarifying disease processes, and microbiology gave a further impetus. Immunology combined microbiology, chemistry, pathology, and physiology to provide even greater explanatory force. When we appreciate all these complex interactions, we no longer can consider an organ as isolated from other organs, nor one bodily function independent of other functions.

Independence, however, is a relative matter. For practical purposes physicians can and do regard certain areas of the body as the site of certain disease processes. Furthermore, particular physiological functions show special correlation with particular diseases. A modern textbook of medicine, in arranging diseases, will provide a rough localization. Thus, a modern text will place renal diseases in one category, cardiovascular diseases in another. This categorization goes not so much by single organs as by systems—certain organs seem to work together as a more or less functional entity and thus can offer a locus for individual diseases.

With such a schema we would say that this disease has its locus in the hematopoietic system, that one in the respiratory system. A further subdivision was well recognized from antiquity. The distinction that the classical authors made between *idiopathic* and *sympathic* corresponds to our distinction of primary and secondary. A disease that originated in a particular organ was idiopathic. A disease that originated in one organ and attacked another organ later, produced a sympathic ailment.

Despite these widespread usages, we must have grave doubts regarding the alleged site or primacy of a disease. The concepts may suffice for practical purposes, but break down when we consider marginal or unusual cases. Let me point to a few examples. A woman had cancer of the breast. At operation the breast and axillary lymph nodes were removed and she remained well for eighteen years. Then she showed evidence of a mass in the abdomen, and surgical exploration showed a well circumscribed tumor mass involving the root of the bowel. This tumor, in its microscopic appearance, was identical with that of the breast, removed eighteen years previously. The pathologist had no hesitation in diagnosing carcinoma metastatic from the breast. Presumably some cancer cells had escaped from the original tumor, settled in the mesentery, and lain dormant for about fifteen to seventeen years. Then these cancer cells had started to grow again. If now we ask, "Where was the disease?" we have an interesting problem.

In one sense the metastatic disease had its site in a mesenteric lymph node. But we cannot ignore the important phenomenon that the cells had lain dormant until something led to renewed growth. What had inhibited the growth potential? How and why was the inhibition removed? Had some positive stimulus overcome the inhibitory factors operative until then? Clearly, we do not know, but the mechanism, whatever it might be, plays an important part in the disease entity. We can be sure that the disease process involves more than the affected lymph node. Since we do not know the mechanism, we cannot identify its locus. We must assume various interactions and various loci, before we can answer the question, "Where is the disease?"

A comparable example would be a woman who had a pigmented spot on her shoulder for at least twenty years. When she became pregnant the pigmented spot rapidly transformed into a malignant melanoma. We know that hormones of pregnancy can have a profound influence on some pigmented lesions, but we do not know how. We must implicate some functional relationship. It would be quite absurd to say that the *disease* is in the skin. We can only say that the obvious clinical manifestations are in the skin.

I will mention two other examples: first, the well-known carrier state in typhoid fever. A food handler or cook who had typhoid fever made an apparently complete clinical recovery, with no residual subjective symptoms of disease. Yet in her gall bladder she continued to harbor typhoid bacilli that passed into the bowel and feces. She spread the disease wherever she worked. Surgical removal of the gall bladder removed the source of the infection. We obviously cannot say that the disease was in the gall bladder. Presumably there was a disturbance of the immune mechanisms, whereby the supposed recovery from typhoid took a form different from the usual course. The bacteria persisted, despite the absence of clinical symptoms. Where, we may appropriately ask, is the disease?

Huntington's chorea is a hereditary condition in which there occurs degeneration of certain portions of the brain, coupled with choreiform movements and mental deterioration. The disease is transmitted by a single dominant autosomal gene. The clinical findings, however, do not become manifest until the patient is in his forties or fifties. Since the clinical manifestations come on rather late in life, the patient may have transmitted the disease to his children before anyone knew that he had that disease.

Before the symptoms became apparent, where was the disease? And when did it start? Is it in the brain? And if so, when did it get there? Should we say that the disease existed from the moment of conception or only when the particular gene exerted its activity during cell division? There is no way of answering these questions and any attempted answer would be arbitrary. These examples suffice to show the limitations of any "seat of disease."

The early physicians recognized the category, diseases of the whole body, distinct from conditions that localized in a particular organ. I suggest that almost every disease affects the whole body. A more particular localization might be useful as a practical device, but it is not really true.

## What Is the Disease? The Problem of Ontology

In Chapter 7, when I discussed some differences between a disease and a clinical entity, I used the word "entity" to mean anything that could serve as a subject of discourse. Now, however, I want to broaden the context.

The word "entity" comes from *ens*, derived in turn from *esse*, to be. This has a gamut of meanings that we can divide into the linguistic and the existential. The formal logic developed by Aristotle deals with linguistic aspects, especially the complex relations of subject and predicate, mediated through the copula *is* (or *are*). Aristotle's discussion of these relations, and of the "categories" and the "predicables," is supremely important not only in logic but in the whole history of thought and in the development of science (including medicine). Some of the Aristotelian distinctions we have already encountered in Chapter 6, on

Classification. I will not, however, discuss further these logical aspects.[7]

The second aspect of *to be* pertains to existence and belongs to that branch of philosophy called ontology—the science of being. Ontology comes from the Greek *on*, from *einai*, to be. If we say that ontology deals with entities, we link the Greek and Latin roots.

Existence implies reality, but, since there are grades of reality, the philosophers want to identify the "really real" or self-subsistent, whose existence does not depend on something else. Dependence would indicate merely a secondary or derivative reality. We see this distinction clearly if we compare rival metaphysical theories. In one ancient school of thought, the basic components of reality were the four qualities—the hot, the cold, the moist, and the dry—called the "primary" qualities, on whose proportions and interactions all other properties, all objects, all activities, depended.

On the other hand, the atomistic philosophy, especially as developed in the 17th century, regarded the atoms as primary and really real, while the four qualities were merely derivative or secondary, dependent on the particular configuration of these atoms. The qualities, thus demoted from their primary status, were called "secondary." What was regarded as primary, and real or self-subsistent in one philosophy, was considered as merely derivative in the other.

This relationship between primary reality and secondary or derivative reality had a strong influence on the notions of disease. The problem is still moot today. For example, we have the widely quoted statement, "There are no diseases but only sick patients." The significance of this glib assertion obviously depends on the meaning attached to the word "are." The statement tells us that, whereas individual patients are real, what we call a disease is only an abstraction and, as a mental construct, merely derivative. We can talk about a disease and regard it as a linguistic entity. This can provide meaningful discourse but does not have "real" existence. Disease would not be really real, but always secondary to the specific individual sick patient.

This distinction, however anemic it may seem today, has engendered passionate argument that relates to the disputes between nominalists and realists. Do general terms, like horse, or red, or disease, have real existence? Platonic philosophy answered in the affirmative and the proponents eventually came to be known as realists. The contrary school of thought, the nominalists, denied any primary reality to these terms but regarded them as mere verbalisms, abstractions, *flatus vocis*. Real existence inhered not in the abstraction but only in the individual, i.e., the particular horse or red object or sick person.

In medicine this dispute had a rather special nomenclature. When we have a group of patients with, say, tuberculosis, is the disease from which they suffer some sort of entity in its own right, distinct from the individual patients? Anyone who answered in the affirmative was an ontologist, who asserted the "real" existence of diseases. The doctrine was strongly opposed by the "physiological school," which stressed the individual reactions of the patient and his interactions with the environment. These anti-ontologists embraced the nominalist position that the alleged disease entity was only an abstraction, a mere name.

The disputes about ontology have produced a considerable literature. The important studies of Rather, Temkin, Pagel, and Niebyl give us an overview as well as important further references. [8]

I approach this problem of ontology indirectly, through a personal recollection. In the mid-1920s I saw a variety show, one act of which has remained vivid in my memory. The curtain rose on a stage totally dark, as if covered with thick black velvet. Subdued music was heard. Suddenly a luminescent hand, isolated and totally disembodied, appeared out of nowhere, moved around, and then disappeared. It reappeared and then other hands, equally luminescent, equally disembodied, became visible. They joined and separated, disappeared and reappeared, performed various rhythmic gyrations. Then disembodied luminescent feet joined the dance. The hands and feet always remained separate objects, and no connection between them could be seen at any time. Then, after suitable rhythmic convolutions all luminescence vanished and the curtain came down on total darkness.

Naturally, the audience wondered how it was done. Perhaps the dancers were completely clad in black but wore gloves and slippers that would fluoresce in so-called "black light." Perhaps the gloves were coated on only one side, so that merely turning the hand or placing it behind the back could bring about disappearance. Perhaps the stage had an apron of black velvet that concealed the slippers until the dancers moved upstage. However, the precise technique is not important for our purpose. I would emphasize, instead, the relationship between what the audience actually saw and what it inferred. What we actually saw—the apparently isolated hands and feet—we call phenomena, directly experienced. We took for granted a connection between these visible objects—the hands and feet—and something else that we could not see, namely a body, whose existence we assumed despite its invisibility, and of whose reality we had no doubt.

The older philosophers would regard this invisible body as "substance," as a unifying but invisible substrate for what was actually perceived. In this sense "substance," although not itself perceived, provided a unity that rendered experience orderly. For the phenomena observed on the stage the "substance" would be a human body. This gives coherence to the phenomena, provides a suitable agency and causal relationships, and furnishes at least a partial explanation that makes the observations intelligible. Many causal factors we can only guess at, such as special gloves and slippers, and a special "light" source. But the concept of a human body, inferred but not observed, brings order into our experience. Such a body, even though we do not see it, we regard as fully real and in no sense a *flatus vocis*.

At this point I would draw a comparison between the stage performance just discussed and a disease. In both instances we first of all describe what we see. On the stage there are the fluorescing hands and feet, isolated, apparently discrete, yet creating an orderly rhythmic pattern. In a disease we have various symptoms—fever, cough, low white cell count, increased sedimentation rate, cavitation of the lung, and the like.[9] Just as the movements of isolated luminescent hands and feet are not self-subsistent, so too the symptoms are considered equally not self-subsistent. Just as we inferred an entity that unifies the seemingly disparate motions of the limbs, so too we infer some entity that unifies the symptoms. In both cases the manifestations are not independent. They depend on something more basic, more real, that gives them a coherence. This real something, whatever it might prove to be, would have a primary status to which the manifestations would be secondary.

But for disease, what *is* that primary entity that underlies the symptoms and provides them with order and unity? Medical history gives us a succession of answers, among which I would mention such terms as the "substantial form" or the "archeus." These earlier views I have discussed at length in other books[10] to which I would refer the reader who wants details. Here I will emphasize two factors. The alleged entity that underlay the symptoms was regarded as fully real. It was also fully immaterial. If this conjunction strikes the reader as strange, he need only think of the concept of soul. In religious philosophy the soul is both real and immaterial. But immaterial reality was not restricted to religious concepts. In medicine the existence of immaterial real entities was the essence of the neogalenic philosophy. It was a major aspect of medical science, that permeated the Paracelsian-Helmontian thinking, the doctrines of Stahl and the vitalism of the 18th and 19th centuries. One influential doctrine held that disease was a "parasite" attacking the body, which tried to defend itself. While other views were more objective, all would reject the dictum that only sick patients were real. On the contrary, the disease was also real.

The scientific revolution that had its big impetus in the 17th century dampened scientific interest in immaterial entities and directed attention to what could be observed, weighed, and measured. Such concepts as soul, archeus, and immaterial substance were extruded from science and shunted over to religion or to mysticism. In the resulting intellectual climate the nominalist position could prevail: immaterial entities like substantial forms were not real but mere verbal entities, *flatus vocis* abstracted from something truly real.

In both my examples—the isolated luminescent hands and feet and the symptoms of disease—I indicated the need for "something" that underlay the phenomena and provided a unity. In the stage performance the entity behind the phenomena was a human body, which comes within the rubric of science—real, material, three-dimensional, with parts that might be directly observed and measured. In diseases, however, substantial forms and archei had lost their standing in science so that the older ontology was rendered untenable. A new ontology with a materialistic base began to emerge. The entity behind the disease symptoms was asserted to be something material, something observable and measurable.

This shift resulted from the scientific advances of the 19th century, especially in microscopy and later in bacteriology. Rudolph Virchow exemplified the trend. Whereas in his earlier years he violently opposed the traditional ontology, he later changed his mind so that he finally equated disease with what was directly observable. He declared, "The disease entity is an altered body-part, or, expressed in first principles, an altered cell or aggregate of cells, whether tissue or organ."[11] Disease for him thus *was* the morphologic changes in tissues. Here, at last, was something that physicians might point to.

Unfortunately, among the other defects of this view, the changes observable under the microscope are in large part nonspecific. Inflammation or caseation or atrophy can appear in a wide variety of diseases. Virchow neglected the essence of ontology, namely, specificity. Wherein lay this specificity? No single tissue change could furnish an answer. The discovery of bacteria gave a slight encouragement to the materialistic ontology. When physicians could point to a bacterium, they thought, for a brief spell, that they were pointing to *the* disease, but disillusionment came speedily. Even for infectious diseases, bacteria were only one limiting or causal factor. Other factors were equally important, as the early immunologists quickly realized. And the non-infectious diseases had no connection with bacteria.

For the ontologist the disease, in some way, is a dynamic unity, a process with a time course and a specificity. Even though different patients may have quite varied manifestations, the unity permits recognition and identification. What is it that provides the unity and specificity? Pointing to tissue changes or to bacteria was not an adequate answer.

For the modern ontologist the unifying factor is some definite pattern or set of relationships. In earlier chapters I have already indicated that disease is a pattern. Hence our problem boils down to the question, "How *real* is a pattern?" Can it constitute a primary entity, truly real, or is it always secondary?

These questions were implicit in the work of Robert Boyle, who in the 17th century helped to achieve the triumph of the mechanical philosophy, with corresponding decline in the Galenic thought modes. For Boyle, as subsequently for John Locke, the atoms were real, and the four "primary" qualities—the hot, cold, moist, and dry—resulted from a particular arrangement of the atoms. In a loose terminology, configurations of atoms *caused* the hot, cold, moist, and dry; hence these were secondary to the configurations.

Yet Boyle had to characterize the atoms in some way, and in his voluminous writings he indicated four properties that he regarded as the truly primary qualities, namely, size, shape, motion, and "texture" or pattern. To be an atom meant to have size and shape, to possess motion, and to participate in an arrangement. These properties which he attributed to atoms—the size, shape, motion and texture—were not *caused* by the atoms but helped to *constitute* the atoms.[12]

However, of these four properties, pattern or texture is different from the others. Whereas size and shape and motion might characterize a single atom, pattern involves a relationship to other atoms. The pattern remains distinct from the components that enter into it. Patterns or texture correspond in a rough way to the Universals of Plato or (after we make due allowances for the differences between Plato and Aristotle) to the Aristotelian Form. After explicitly rejecting this, Boyle had covertly smuggled it back into his own philosophy—a fine example of the popular statement that what you push out through the door comes back through the window.

Form, pattern, or relationship remain an essential aspect of reality just as much today as in the time of Aristotle or Boyle. In current thinking we need only mention isomers in chemistry. The same atoms, when placed in a different order, may give a totally different result. The arrangement is the crucial feature. In stereo-isomerism the structure is the same but the relationships exhibit a mirror-image, again producing a distinguishable and specific product.

How "real" is arrangement or relationship? Of course, merely asserting a relationship means little. The modern ontologist still has the task of establishing that relationship, demonstrating that it does in some way reflect reality. The task is arduous—finding the constancy of relationship that persists among the different and variable concrete examples. We are dealing with the age-old problem of the uniformity or unity among manifest differences, a problem that engages the modern scientist just as much as it did Plato. The modern scientist can wholeheartedly subscribe to Platonic doctrine. Today, just as was the case twenty-four hundred years ago, the investigator who perceives an inner connection among phenomena will not "rest contented with the manifold diversities which are seen in a multitude of things until he has comprehended all of them that have any affinity within the bounds of one similarity and embraced them within the reality of a single kind."[13] He seeks the unity that underlies apparent diversity. This unity he finds in pattern and relationship, somehow more basic than the individuals originally observed.

Despite the changes in our intellectual climate, the so-called problem of universals is as significant today as in 400 B.C. We need not imagine a heavenly realm of disembodied forms subsisting in the mind of God or constituting a mystical Good. We can accept the concept that form (or pattern or relationship) are "immaterial," and that form and matter are inseparable. Yet in that combination we must distinguish patterns or relationships and assign them full reality.

Establishing a relationship can be arduous and difficult. At any time an alleged pattern may become unacceptable through new knowledge. In such a case we do not deny the reality of patterns but only that we have not yet acquired insight into the real relationship. In disease, of course, the relationships that we *assert* are continuously changing, as Chapter 2 adequately describes.

Any disease, however convincingly asserted as an entity, does not necessarily mirror reality but only approaches it. We accept a pattern as real—i.e., that of which we must take account—as long as it remains harmonious with other experience.[14] To pursue this line of thought would carry us far into epistemology and metaphysics, which may hold little interest for most readers. I would emphasize only that *patterns are an inseparable and primary part of whatever we call reality*; that, like the substantial form of the neogalenic physicians, pattern is "immaterial"; and that we must at all times have great humility in asserting that any given pattern is real. All such assertions are tentative. To say that something is real has meaning only with the proviso, "subject to further experience that may change our views."

Today the questions, when, where, and what is the disease? if conscientiously examined, cement our connection with our medical past. The answers have changed, but the problems have not.

*CAUSE*

———————◗ ◖———————

## CHAPTER 9

# The Causes of Disease: I

*One of the busiest words in English* is the monosyllable "cause." The word itself and the ideas behind it lurk almost everywhere—in everyday activities, in medicine, law, history, philosophy, sociology, economics, in virtually every intellectual and practical pursuit. However, the meaning and implications will vary according to context. Although we are here concerned primarily with medicine, we cannot study causation without briefly surveying some of the different meanings that we find in other disciplines.

Let us look at a few examples. A minute cinder blew into your eye, and produced great pain, redness, and tearing. Rubbing the eye did no good. You went to the physician, who skillfully turned back the upper lid and removed a minute speck. In everyday language the cinder was the cause of the disease, and removing the cinder cured the disease.

You switch on the lamp. The light flashes momentarily and then goes out. You say there is a short circuit, and you go through a variety of procedures to find out where it might be. You finally locate a place in the wiring where the insulation was eroded and two bare wires came into contact. The break in the insulation caused the short circuit.

Such usages represent ordinary common sense, and offer no complications. But most situations are not quite so simple. Take another example. A building has caught fire and burns. What was the cause of the fire? The insurance company and the police want to know whether there was arson. The fire department, in addition, wants to know whether there were building-code violations. Investigations showed that the electric wiring was defective, the sprinkler system did not function properly, and there were numerous violations of the building code. But there was also clear evidence of arson.

Here we have a multiplicity of factors, some more relevant than others. Although the wiring was defective, there was no evidence that it had anything to do with starting the blaze. This was initiated by the deliberate activities of an arsonist. Nevertheless, the building-code violations and the failure of the sprinkler system undoubtedly contributed to the spread of the fire.

In a situation such as this we must be quite precise in the question that we ask. "What caused the fire?" is quite different from "What caused the house to burn?" The former permits a simple common-sense answer: the arsonist set it. The latter question involves contributory factors and accessory conditions; common sense is no longer such a reliable or "obvious" guide.

There is one further answer that we can offer. The fire started because the temperature rose until it reached the combustion point. Let us assume that this is 600 degrees. Then we could say, "The fire started (or the house burned) because, in the presence of oxygen, the temperature rose to 600 degrees." An investigator would say, "True, but irrelevant." I think we would all agree, but we can legitimately ask the question, "Why is it irrelevant?" And here we glimpse our first major complication in trying to understand causation.

The combustion point and its accurate definition are matters of science, which, in this instance, propounds a generalization, applicable to a class of objects (let us say, the class of seasoned soft pine wood). The arson investigation, on the other hand, is concerned not with scientific generalization, but with a specific incident at a definite time and place. Involved is a singular event, unique and never to be repeated in all its circumstances. The question that needs to be answered is not, "Why did the house burn?" but rather, "Why, of all the houses in the community, did *this* house catch fire?" And to say that the combustion point of soft pine is 600 degrees does not answer that question.

I regard any specific incident, any concrete event, as an aspect of *history*. We may think that only such important events as the crowning of Charlemagne, or the discovery of America, should be called history. But we must also include the setting afire of a modest dwelling in a depressed neighborhood. History deals with individual events, in contrast to science, which deals with classes, generalizations, and abstractions.

We create classes by selecting from several individuals the properties that interest us. This is abstraction, another word for selectively ignoring certain other properties as not important for the questions we want answered. What we ignore will vary according to the subject matter and to the interests involved. But common to all classes in science is one supremely important feature: absence of that unique particularity which comprises the essence of history.

A further example will illustrate additional points important for later analysis of causation in medicine. Imagine an airplane crash. The investigation attributed the fault to the control tower: one person had not been sufficiently alert. "Human error" on the part of this particular person was considered the cause of the accident.

The investigators probed further. Why did the man in the control tower make that error at that particular time? Study brought to light several important facts. The man had had a quarrel with his wife that very morning and was "upset." For many months past he had been tense and irritable and under the care of a psychiatrist. The psychiatrist had uncovered evidence of neurotic personality with a strong mother fixation that prevented him from making a good marital adjustment. And this fixation, in turn, was traced back to childhood experiences.

Here we have an unbroken chain of causal factors that came to a focus in the control tower and led to the failure in performance and to the resulting crash. Can we say that the cause of the crash was the mother fixation of the controller, leading to a neurotic personality, precipitating a quarrel that clouded his judgment, and that this in turn resulted in the crash?

No judge or jury would say that the cause of the crash was the long-buried childhood experiences. Any such connection seems too tenuous and remote. Thus we come up against the problem of relevance. How do we decide whether a given factor is "sufficiently" relevant to be deemed a causal link? *What* is relevant in determining responsibility? This is a basic aspect of causation, most urgent, perhaps, in the law,[1] but applicable to medicine as well; and when we have achieved an answer, we face the further questions: *how* relevant? how should various factors be evaluated? No two persons will give the same answers, and that is why historians differ. From this we must conclude that judgments of relevance depend on the individual and on the context. We will find this as true in medicine as in political science or economics.

Before proceeding to specifically medical contexts, I would emphasize a few general points derived from these examples. The meaning of cause will vary according to the situation. The common-sense or everyday usage is simplistic. It deals with "the" cause, as a singular term. Sometimes "the" cause is deemed part of a linear series, like a row of dominoes. If the earlier member of the series is set into motion, it will successively affect the next in a chain reaction, culminating in the final "effect." We often speak of this as a "causal chain," implying a succession of individual links. We should instead think of causation in a broader fashion, as a congeries of factors resembling a network rather than a chain.

I emphasize strongly that statements about a singular event differ from statements about a class. Classes, products of abstraction, are the domain of science. In contrast, singular or unique events form the province of history, in its broad sense. I stress also the importance of relevance in any causal relationship. Is *this* bit of information relevant to the problem we are trying to solve? And here is the area where disagreement chiefly prevails among the various seekers after truth.

## II

Medicine is not in any way a unit. It serves functions both practical and theoretical. The former involves taking care of the sick patient, who ordinarily presents considerable urgency. The doctor must *do* something, and often do it quickly. And, even if the time factor is extended by days or weeks, urgency still remains. Help too long delayed ceases to be help. On the other hand, medicine is also a part of biological science, which, like all science, is timeless. Truth is patient, even though sometimes a special urgency affects individual scientists—e.g., the haste to develop an atom bomb before the enemy does so; or to decipher the genetic code ahead of any rival team. But these do not affect the essential timelessness of science.

The search for causes is perhaps the essence of science. Aristotle had already made this abundantly clear. The empiric, he pointed out, does not have any knowledge of causes. He knows *that* a thing is so, but he does not know *why* it is so. He learns by experience. On the other hand, the person whom we would designate as a man of science knows the *why* of things. He had command of theory. He knows not merely the "particulars" but the "universals." The man of experience knows that fire is hot, but the man of science knows why it is hot.

Daniel Sennert, perhaps the leading neogalenic physician in the 17th century, expressed this view clearly. *Cum scire sit rem per caussam cognoscere. Scire*, to know, is the root of our word science, and we could translate the passage, in a free manner, as "Science consists in knowing things by their causes." A more literal rendition would be, "To know scientifically is to understand things through their causes." Or, a little more freely, "To have scientific knowledge is to understand the causes of things."[2]

The distinction between knowing things by their causes and knowing them through practical experience applies to quite varied activities. The farmer, through experience, has learned what and when to plant, how to care for his crop, and when to harvest. But he does not know why he does these things rather than something else, except for the simple answer, "It works." On the other hand, the devotee of scientific farming knows why, and can get improved yields through knowledge of causes.

In medicine the empiric treats the patient without knowing the causes. He expects that what has helped in the past will help in the future. If he has had good training, his experience will probably make him a reliable practitioner; poor training will

make him unreliable. But in either case he is contented with
what works and does not worry about the theory. The scientific
physician, as the man of knowledge, wants to know the why of
things and he uses this knowledge of causes when he treats the
patient. He tries first to discover and then to attack the causes
of the disease. Today we devote much of our medical education
to inculcating the students with this ideal, but we must remember that the very same situation and the same ideal prevailed in
past times as well as in the present.

The history of medicine reveals the many different causes that
have been propounded to explain disease. The leading physicians, of whatever era, offered treatment that accorded with
their theories, and these reflected the prevalent notions of cause.
But theories conflict; explanations change; concepts of cause vary
from one era to another. When we ask, "What is the cause of
this patient's disease?" the answer must have the preamble, "It
depends on whom you ask."

Traditionally, the "cause" of disease can refer to either of two
quite distinct possibilities—something concrete or something abstract. A concrete object we can point to, perhaps handle and
manipulate—the cinder in the eye that caused the conjunctivitis;
or the stone in the common duct that caused colic and jaundice;
or the inflamed appendix, responsible for the severe bellyache.
The surgeon brings about a cure by removing these objects. He
probably has no doubt that these concrete entities, visible and
palpable, are truly the cause of the ailments.

Let us now go back to early Greek medicine, when the humors and their relationships were thought to determine health
and disease. In classical theory there were four primary humors:
the blood, phlegm, yellow bile, and black bile. Health consisted
in the "proper" proportion among them, and disproportion resulted in disease. In certain cases the patient could readily appreciate that something was present in excess. His nose might
drip mucus or he might have a watery diarrhea, or he might
have an edema where his ankles swelled with obvious excess of
fluid. These findings harmonize readily with the cinder or the
gallstone—something visible and tangible that shouldn't be
there.

Suppose you wanted to continue the search. The gallstone caused a disease, but what caused the gallstone? Excess phlegm caused the diarrhea or the coryza, but what caused the excess phlegm? Here we get into a quite different area of thought. When we try to give causes of causes, we soon leave behind anything that we can see and feel and fall back on abstractions, on conceptual entities like a disproportion and coction, for the Greeks, or, for present-day medicine, on cholesterol metabolism and the complexities of liver function. In ancient and modern medicine alike we would be leaving the realm of the concrete to rely on the abstract.

Abstractions (or relationships) we cannot see. They are conceptual entities, the products of reason, requiring mental activity for their creation and mental activity for their appreciation. In abstraction we engage in a process of selection. We progressively discard more and more properties, until we are left with a residue, abstracted from the infinite richness of the individual entities. When we manipulate the abstractions in appropriate fashion, compare them, display their relationships, and draw conclusions from these relationships, we are creating theories.

Conceptual entities, embedded in theories, were regarded as causes. Boerhaave, who carefully articulated a systematic presentation, provides an especially good example. Since limited technology restricted his powers of direct observation, his concepts of finer structure were derived through reasoning. The body he regarded as composed of solids and fluids. The ultimate component of the solids were elementary particles that combined to form fibers. The fluids consisted of various humors, whose ultimate constituents were also minute particles. His system thus rested on a modified atomistic hypothesis.[3]

The body functioned according to principles of mechanics and hydraulics, powered by the circulation and by the interaction of mechanical forces. In addition, Boerhaave, as an eclectic, adopted certain chemical concepts of acids and alkalis and "glutens" and similar terms related to chemistry of the day. These various terms represented inference, not observation. They began, however, as concrete observations on a simple level and then, through a process of abstraction, elaboration, and combination, were built up into a system of abstract entities that we call theory.

Boerhaave explained diseases by various causal mechanisms related to the basic principles. There were diseases of the solids and diseases of the fluids. The diseases of the solids fell into two main types, depending on whether the elemental fibers were too stiff or too lax. Too great a stiffness, for example, "causes the vessels, which consist of these fibers, to be less flexible, narrower, and shorter . . . with all the consequences following hereupon." Other kinds of disease would arise if fibers were too lax. The fluids could also give rise to disease. They might exhibit acid or alkaline "acrimonies." The acid acrimony, for example, "produces sour belchings, hunger, heart-burning, iliac pains, flatulencies, inactivity of the bile . . . acid chyle, and excrements with sour smell. These are its effects in the stomach and intestines."[4]

Boerhaave used the Latin terms *facit* and *producit* to convey the causal relationship between the altered fibers or humours and the symptoms of disease. Thus, *the concepts that he used as the basic explanatory principles he also regarded as the causes of disease.* He described—i.e., he hypothesized—in considerable detail the ways in which these fibers or fluids might be affected by environmental or internal disturbances and thereby was offering causes of causes. He did not differentiate between the objects that he could see and those whose existence he inferred, but both classes participated in the causal nexus. Concrete environmental factors he could observe directly. These affected the hypothetical or conceptual fibers and fluid particles whose existence he inferred, and these, when altered, Boerhaave considered as the real causes of those anatomical and functional changes that characterized disease. Causality for him thus involved an interaction between concrete and hypothetical entities.

## III

*Correlation*

David Hume emphasized that we never perceive causation as a datum of experience—we perceive only sequences and conjunc-

tions. One type of conjunction is correlation. We see this especially well in the writings of Hippocrates. His great fame rests
not on any theories that he elaborated but on his descriptions
and correlations. Many of his descriptions are so vivid that today, twenty-five-hundred years later, we have no difficulty in
making a modern diagnosis. We also have the simple generalizations that assert a togetherness of events, that phenomenon A
is associated with phenomenon B. They belong together, in a
fashion not specified. This association of phenomena, considered
as a bare togetherness, we call a correlation, a relationship of
some sort not further specified.

There is the explicit statement, "*That* A and B belong together is an assertion of fact." There is no indication *why* they
go together. *That* they relate to each other is an empirical statement. *Why* they relate would be a causal statement, an inferential or rationalistic assertion.

The *Aphorisms* of Hippocrates are among his most famous
and most influential works. They offer descriptions of events
that he observed not once but several times. Out of the total
events he realized that certain features belonged together in a
special relationship. The remaining features of the separate cases
he ignored. In brief pithy statements he asserted the togetherness
as a generalizaton. I will give two examples in paraphrase. Dys-
entery, he said, that starts with the passage of black blood is
fatal. If the breasts of a pregnant woman regress suddenly, she
will soon miscarry.[5]

These two statements—representative of hundreds more—
summarized the personal experience of a keen and busy physician and served as advice for others who might meet with similar cases. The aphorisms, for the most part, carry a future
reference. They tell us what we can expect in the ordinary course
of nature. They have a predictive value, with a high degree of
probability. In modern terms we would say that they have a
high coefficient of correlation.

They do not give any reasons why. They make no effort to
trace any hidden connections between the terms. That such connections existed, no one doubted, for nature was orderly and
reliable. But any attempt at explanation would be speculative.

Speculation was certainly rife among the Greeks, but it was the great glory of Hippocrates, and the basis of his renown in the 17th and 18th centuries, that he had stressed observation, description, and low-level generalization.

In the light of modern medicine we today can see connections between the terms of his correlations. We are not restricted to saying that A and B go together, but we can give reasons why they go together. These connections, hidden from Hippocrates, provide causal explanations.

The passage of blood per rectum was a familiar phenomenon. If the blood were red, it was clearly fresh and presumably due to hemorrhoids. Blood that was black was not fresh but old; it must have derived from bleeding higher in the gastrointestinal tract and remained in the intestine long enough to turn color. Bleeding of this type might, for example, have been due to cancer of the bowel, or to ulcer of the stomach or duodenum, as the most common causes. Today we not only can make a specific diagnosis but can intervene and often cure the patient. The Greeks, who had negligible knowledge of what went on inside the body, could not make any specific diagnosis. Whatever might have produced an internal bleeding they recognized as incurable by the skills they possessed.

Modern medicine explains the bodily changes in pregnancy through a hormonal interaction that we recognize as extremely complex, involving numerous glands and organs. Lactation is such a hormonal effect, where the linkage of events relates directly to a living fetus. Death of the fetus will alter the hormonal production so that the breasts, no longer stimulated, will regress. Since the expulsion of a dead fetus may be delayed, a regression of the breasts can be an early sign that the fetus is not viable, and that the hormonal sequences have been interrupted. Hippocrates, in his *Aphorisms*, did not offer any explanation at all but merely noted the correlation that, as a datum of experience, is still approximately valid today.

Hippocrates did not in any way imply that black blood caused death. Some additional factors would be needed, not mentioned in the aphorism, to supply a causal connection. Similarly, the regression of the breast did not cause the miscarriage, but any assertion of a causal relation would require some additional factors not yet specified. What are these additional factors? There are many possible categories, but for simplicity I will choose only three for special comment. The first I will call the intercalation of causes.

## Intercalation of Causal Factors

Under this heading I will present two instances. The first will be the familiar cinder in the eye. On a windy day the patient feels a sudden flick in the eye, immediately develops some discomfort, and then pain, redness, and tearing. The physician, making a diagnosis of conjunctivitis, removes a minute cinder from beneath the upper lid. My second case: on a picnic nine members of a group ate chicken salad, two others did not. All those who ate the chicken salad became sick with abdominal pain, fever, and diarrhea; the other two had no symptoms.

In each of these instances we assert a direct causal relation between the respective terms—cinder and conjunctivitis, chicken salad and diarrhea. The connections would have been equally clear to physicians and to laymen, whether today or in the time of Sydenham or of Galen.

Scientists would want to know, *how* do we get from cause to effect, from event A to event B? Even the layman knew *that* there was a causal connection, but the scientist wants to know the intermediate steps.

The cinder produced an inflammation, a process that became more complex the more it was studied. It was explicitly described by Celsus in the first century A.D., with its characteristic signs of *dolor*, *tumor*, *rubor*, and *calor*—pain, swelling, redness, and heat. These features comprise what philosophers call a non-random pattern, to be explained "by causal mechanisms, in general unobservable, whose behavior generates the observed pattern."[6] Scientists offered concepts to serve as intermediate steps and thus account for the pattern. The successive concepts of inflammation make a fascinating history but I will mention only one instance. Boerhaave derived his theories from mechanics and hydraulics. Since he knew nothing of our modern cell theory, he explained inflammation by two factors, an obstruction of minute vessels and an increased force of the circulation. The obstruction might result, e.g., from minute particles getting wedged into extremely minute vessels and getting impacted by the increased force of the blood.[7]

In the 19th century improved microscopy and the emergence of cell theory introduced new factors that made Boerhaave's concepts untenable. Pathologists had at their command abundant new data—various blood and tissue cells, phagocytosis, blood vessel changes, diapedesis, exudation, necrosis, and numerous other changes that they could see under the microscope. These observations led to new concepts such as chemotaxis, enzymes, behavior of plasma proteins, specific properties of tissue breakdown, to name but a few. All of them had causal relevance. The study of inflammation in its observational and theoretical concepts became enormously complex. The medical student learns only the major outlines of the theories, whose esoteric details are reserved for specialized monographs and for highly technical papers.

The whole theory of inflammation, constantly expanding like the universe, can be intercalated between terms A and B, between "the" cause (the cinder) and "the" effect (the full-blown inflammation). Most physicians do not know the details, and usually do not care. They know the beginning and the end of the sequence, and know that *someone* can provide a step-wise progression of the intermediate events.

The second example, that "bad" food produced illness, was also familiar from earliest times. The early physicians were fully aware that various environmental factors, including food and drink, might cause disease. The designation "non-naturals"[8] specified some of the categories that could affect the state of health. Besides the ingested substances the list included the air we breathe, the excreta and retenta, motion and rest, sleep and wakefulness, and passions of the mind. Scientists propounded a succession of theories to explain *how* the causal connection took place.

Theories changed as knowledge increased. Ferments and acrids, quite satisfactory at one time, gave way to more precise concepts of bacterial infection. The isolation of different kinds of bacteria, the knowledge of toxins, the reactions between the bacteria and the host, the knowledge of immunology, all contributed to complex theories of infection that could be intercalated between eating the chicken salad and getting sick.

In these examples (which could be multiplied indefinitely) scientists have sought hidden links in the causal relation and have offered theories, some excellently grounded in facts, others more speculative. To explain the connection between A and B, between, say, "bad" food and diarrhea, concepts became progressively more explicit and showed increasingly complex details. A primitive explanation might be "imbalance of humors with excess of phlegm." More specific would be "poison," with its own broad sphere of relationship. Still more explicit is "acrid," which has detailed relationship to specific chemical phenomena. "Bacteria" bring in much greater complexity. Staphylococcus, Salmonella, and Shigella are a few of the possible offenders, but different bacteria act in different ways. Was a toxin involved? If so, was it produced in the food before ingestion or only after the bacteria were swallowed? Or perhaps no toxin was acting, but the diarrhea resulted from direct invasion of the intestinal mucosa by the bacteria?

If we try to answer the question, "How do we get from A to B?" we face staggering complexities, constantly increasing as scientists discover more data and expand their theories accordingly. The terms of the various theories would be intercalations between A and B.

### Accessory Cause—Concomitant

In the previous examples ordinary usage would say that event A was the cause of event B. Sometimes, however, such a formulation would be obviously too simple. Then, in generalized terms, event A could be regarded as only a partial cause.

Two men are walking down the street. They both stumble on the curb. One man breaks his leg, the other does not. Was the stumble the cause of the fracture? If so, why did not the second man also break his leg? We might say, perhaps, that the second man recovered his balance more effectively, so that the stumble was not as severe. However, when the first man went to the hospital he was found to have a cancer of the lung that had spread to the bone and reduced it to a shell. Although the stumble produced only a minor strain that would have had no effect on normal tissue, in the diseased bone a fracture occurred.

"The" cause of the fracture thus has at least two components. There was a predisposing factor—the severely weakened bone—and the precipitating factor—the actual stumble. They represent co-causes; only together could they cause the fracture.

In a second case a man had a tooth pulled. The bleeding that normally occurs will ordinarily stop spontaneously. In this case, however, the patient continued to bleed until he had to consult a physician. Clearly, pulling the tooth initiated the bleeding but with equal clarity was not the whole cause. Physicians discovered that the patient had a blood disorder, namely, a deficiency in platelets. Pulling the tooth was only a partial cause; the effect—the continued bleeding—depended as well on the predisposing cause—the platelet deficiency.

In disease the problem of partial causes, or coincidental causal factors, was well recognized by Galen. Traditional medicine had the rather formidable adjectives, proegumenical and procatarctic, to indicate the more familiar predisposing and exciting (or occasional) causes. In the examples given, the bone metastases and the platelet disorders are the predisposing causes, the stumble and the tooth-pulling the respective exciting causes.

In reference to disease, the older physicians who followed the Galenic tradition did not speak of *the* cause, without qualification but ordinarily specified the *kind* of cause. Physicians of the 19th and 20th centuries, trying to avoid everything that savored of Galenic foolishness, tended to ignore the important distinctions that earlier physicians had made. Elsewhere I have discussed in considerable detail the older formulation of the causal relationships.[9]

### Accessory Causes—Antecedent

In the first section we studied cases of the type, A caused B. In the next, the formulation would be, A plus X caused B. Now

I would illustrate the formula, X caused A, which caused B. We are dealing with a combination of causes, but the combination is sequential rather than simultaneous. A single example will suffice.

A man has a cerebral hemorrhage and dies within a few hours. For the death certificate the "immediate" cause of death is, clearly, the cerebral hemorrhage. But the death certificate wants to know how that arose. There might have been trauma, or a brain tumor, or an aneurysm, or high-blood pressure. In the present case the hemorrhage was "due" to elevated blood pressure—hypertension. Then the death certificate asks for further information, an additional link in the causal chain. What caused the hypertension? In the present case the patient had had a history of chronic kidney disease—chronic glomerulonephritis. The death certificate would thus read, "*Cause of death*, cerebral hemorrhage *due to* hypertension, *due to* glomerulonephritis."

At this point the death certificate loses interest, but suppose that we want to pursue the chain still farther. We find out, say, that the patient, when a child, had had scarlet fever, which, as a streptococcus infection, often damages the kidneys. On further query we find that he had always had "poor resistance," that he constantly suffered from sore throats and tonsillitis, and that he lived in a damp climate. Further, that he had a sister who had rheumatic heart disease (also causally related to streptococcus infection). Here we find suggestive evidence of a predisposing cause for his illness, a "low resistance," the popular term whose scientific basis rests on immunology. Furthermore, immunologic defects may have some hereditary background. There may possibly be a genetic factor in his death. Where shall we stop answering the question, "Due to"?

In trying to trace the causes, we find not only a direct linear chain that goes back to childhood but also some accessory factors that I call a circumferential network, such as possible hereditary factors, environmental influences that facilitated infection, or exposure to various noxa. None of these would appear on the death certificate, but this does not exclude their relevance. If we were going to fill out a death certificate for Achilles, would we not give as a causal factor that Thetis, when she dipped the infant in the River Styx, failed to immerse the heel by which she held him?

So far we have been discussing instances where, in common speech, "the" cause was known. In certain events—the inflammation of the eye, the fractured leg, the death from apoplexy or drowning—the connection that I have put in the form "A causes B" seems a manifest fact of experience. For the most part, we cease to look farther, but, if we do look farther, we invariably find that our original formulation was too simple and that additional factors, not immediately apparent, have relevance. These additional factors might be conceptual or concrete; they might be intercalated between the apparent cause and its effect; or they might accompany the apparent cause, either simultaneously or successively.

## IV

Any causal assertion that at first glance seems simple and adequate will turn out, on closer study, to have broad ramifications. When in common speech we talk about the cause, these ramifications do not trouble us much, for the practical affairs of life require us to ignore remote connections. But often we want to go farther than the limits imposed by common usage. How far should we go? In pursuing the question, "What is the cause?" we find that the meaning of cause will vary according to the context. Who is asking the question, and for what purpose? How much detail does he want? What sort of answer will satisfy him? Since the same word "cause" is used in different situations, the meaning at any given time may be uncertain. The problems engendered by this uncertainty have produced a literature enormous in extent and complexity.

My discussion so far, centering on medicine, has touched a few of the problems and I have tried to indicate certain points of view. In the study of causation I make a sharp distinction between the singular event—e.g., "Why did *this* patient develop a duodenal ulcer at this time?"—and the generalization—e.g.,

"What is the cause of tuberculosis?" The singular event is the domain of history, the generalizations, of science. The generalizations propounded by science are often regarded as "laws."

In neither the singular event nor the generalization is a single antecedent event a satisfactory answer to the question, "What is the cause?" Neither is a simple linear chain of events. Instead, there is always extensive ramification, backward and sideways, extending indefinitely, although with diminished relevance. Instead of a chain we must think of a network, with interaction of the various factors. There are always co-factors that interact. Some factors will seem more important than others, but *the importance will relate to the interests of the investigator*.

When we think of causal factors we may think of a focus and a periphery. We focus on those factors which we consider the most relevant; the remainder we relegate to the periphery. What comes into focus and what is banished to the periphery will depend on interest and purpose, and may change from time to time. No two investigators will have the same focus, for they will not agree on what they consider the most important.

When we start to talk about the plurality of causes and to clarify the relations that come into play, we must embark on a somewhat different analysis. We must also note in greater detail the differences between the causal relation in history and in science, depending on whether we attend to the individual instance or to the class. These topics I will take up in the next chapter.

———◄ ►———

## CHAPTER 10

# *The Causes of Disease*: II

*Popular usage constantly refers to* one event as *the* cause of another. In this usage, however, the definite article implies something unique, when actually there is multiplicity. We see the fallacy if we look at the officers of a corporation. If there are ten vice-presidents, it would be wrong to call any one of them *the* vice-president. We can, however, achieve accuracy if we add further determinants. It is entirely correct to say, Mr. X. is *the* vice-president in charge of personnel.

We find the same situation in regard to causes. To speak of *the* cause suggests that there is only one, a view that philosophers often call the doctrine of monocausation. This we find, for example, in medical texts that assert, "The cause of typhoid fever is the typhoid bacillus," or in popular essays that maintain that the cause of lowered mortality in pneumonia is the discovery and use of antibiotics.

The monocausationists, of course, realize that the claim does not hold up under even minimal examination, so that the supporters admit grudgingly that other factors should be recognized. A good monocausationist, however, will downgrade these as of secondary importance. *The* cause gets transformed into the important cause, or the major cause, or the one to which we must pay attention. Luckily, this concession opens the door to a better understanding that will take account of context and circumstances.

Aristotle fully realized that the concept of *the* cause, unmodified, had no validity without specification. He greatly clarified the subject by distinguishing his well-known four causes, four distinct contexts or usages, in each of which the term "cause" had a different sense. The sculptor who makes a statue is certainly a cause of the statue. The marble out of which the statue is made is also a cause. But so too is the sitter who was the model of the statue. And we must also include the commission that authorized the statue so that it could be placed in the library—the purpose for which it was created. Aristotle called these the efficient, the material, the formal, and the final causes, respectively. Each referred to some particular facet of the causal relation. They were not interchangeable. Since each relates to a unique set of factors, we may properly speak of *the* cause only when we specify the particular set. The marble, for example, is *a* cause of the statue, but is *the* material cause.

In medicine special attention was directed to what Aristotle called the efficient cause and, in the Galenic tradition, the physicians introduced a vast array of subdivisions that Aristotle had not envisioned. By the 17th century medical writers discriminated a great many different *kinds* of cause, that is, different types of causal relationship, any one of which might be called a causal factor. The physicians used such diverse headings as principal, adjuvant, remote, proximal, external, internal, necessary, contingent, antecedent, conjoint, occasional, continued, and various others as well. These causes differed not only in kind but in importance and degree. There is much overlap, so that we cannot regard the listing as in any way a classification. There is merely a series of categories intended to help us to understand the complexities of the causal relationship, i.e., what I have called the "causal network." For the modern reader, accustomed to monocausation doctrines, the listings tend to confuse rather than to clarify.

When physicians wrote in Latin, there was no confusion. Difficulties arose when Latin texts were rendered into English, for the translators did not pay attention to an important difference between the two languages. Latin does not have any words corresponding to the *a* or *the* of English. In Latin a physician would ask, *"Quod est eius causa?"* which would be literally translated as "What is cause of that?" Since this is not idiomatic English, translators offered, "What is the cause of that?" There is, however, an alternative rendition that is equally accurate but has a very different meaning in English, namely, "What is *a* cause of that?" The definite article, which implies a univocal relationship, would be appropriately used only with some specification, as, *the* antecedent cause, *the* necessary cause, and the like.

On the other hand, the notion of cause could also be regarded in a completely comprehensive fashion, to embrace in a single unity *all* the subdivisions. This usage was well expressed by Lazar Riverius in the 17th century: "This is the most general definition, or rather explication, of morbific cause, which cannot deviate [*alia esse non potuit*] if it is going to embrace all the causes that are considered in medicine." In this preliminary statement I would direct attention to the use of cause—*the* cause—as a singular. It indicates the *totality* of subordinate (and specific) causal factors, i.e., of causes in the plural. Riverius went on, "All those things are given the name of causes which contribute anything to the production of disease, in any way whatever, whether per se or by accident, mediately or immediately [directly or indirectly], or maintain or exacerbate the disease, or affect it in any other way at all."[1]

This broad definition indicates a totality, the aggregate of everything that affects the disease state in any way. We might have trouble in deciding what the definition excludes. Is there anything that has *no relevance at all* to any given phenomenon? We might, perhaps, say that when a man has broken his leg the eclipse of the moon was totally irrelevant. But a firm believer in astrology need not concur. We draw the limits of relevance partly on the basis of common sense, partly on practical considerations, and partly on ignorance. Each generation changes its notion of relevance, to keep pace with changes in the intellectual environment. At present the modern studies in ecology are exerting a great influence on our concepts of relevance.

The concept that the *totality* of causal factors constitutes *the* cause of a given event has remained vigorous and influential. Boerhaave had adopted a variant of this view in the 18th century, and in the 19th century John Stuart Mill expressed himself clearly and forcefully on the subject: "The cause, then, philosophically speaking, is the sum total of the conditions, positive and negative taken together; the whole of the contingencies of every description, which being realized, the consequent invariably follows."[2]

## II

Before discussing the totality of individual factors, we must first study some of the interrelations between the different kinds of causal factors that had been separately enumerated. The 17th-century physicians identified different types of cause, although with considerable overlap, but offered no rigorous definitions that could clearly distinguish one from another. By the mid-18th century the numerous causal factors previously enumerated had been reduced to a few main types. One, the contrast between the predisposing and the precipitating factors, has already been mentioned. In my example I referred to a man with metastatic tumor in his femur, who broke his leg after a minor trauma. The main category, however, the one that has resulted in the most confusion, and the one with which I will deal here, has to do with the terms "remote" and "proximal" causes. With these, unfortunately, we find ambiguity, for both of these terms have a dual usage—an obvious temporal reference and also a usage that I will designate as logical.

The temporal reference is quite easy. Any relevant factor that precedes a particular effect would be a remote cause. Suppose that a man has just had a coronary thrombosis. If we learn that twenty years earlier he had had rheumatic fever, with resulting valvular damage and enlargement of the heart, this would be called a remote cause of the present heart attack. If, moreover, a week ago he lost his job and was under great emotional stress, this too would be a remote cause, but less remote—and hence more proximal—than the attack twenty years ago. In this sense, proximal and remote merely indicate the relative positions on a time scale.

In a causal sequence we ordinarily consider the effect to be the terminus of the causal factors. But this apparently simple statement conceals certain difficulties. Let me give two examples.

Let us imagine a baseball game. The score is tied and the home team is at bat in the last of the ninth. There are none out. The first batter hits a home run and thereby wins the game. The newspaper reporter might say that batter X won the game in the last of the ninth. The logician might say that the home run was *the* proximal cause of the win, for that run was the event that *immediately* preceded the effect. The instant the batter touched the home plate, the game was over. Between touching the home plate and the winning of the game it is not possible to intercalate any additional factor. Stepping on the home plate after satisfying the necessary conditions was the ultimate proximal cause. There was an instantaneous merging of this cause with the effect.

Strictly speaking, hitting the ball over the fence did not win the game but was only a remote cause, getting closer and closer to the effect. With a little ingenuity we can think of other factors that might still have intervened. Suppose that as the runner passed third base he suddenly dropped dead, and never did complete the circuit. The game would not be won. The effect would not have come to pass. *The* proximal cause was stepping on the home plate after touching the other bases.

Every play in the game, prior to the actual touching of the plate, was a remote cause of the win, at different temporal periods removed from the final outcome. In the seventh inning the pitcher struck out all three opposing batters. This was a remote cause, more proximal than the double play in the sixth. But all of these remote causes, individually and in the aggregate, differ from *the* proximal cause, for only in the latter was there any absolute necessity. Between any of the remote causes and the final effect, some additional factor might have intervened to prevent the effect. But *the* proximal cause permits no intervening factor. The necessity is absolute.

There is a special and peculiar relationship between the effect and one particular factor that we call *the* proximal cause. This relationship does not obtain with any remote cause. Let us examine this peculiar relationship further. I will give another example, originally offered by Herman Boerhaave in the 18th century. He pointed to a balance. On one side was a weight of 100 pounds, on the other, 99 pounds. If we now add exactly one pound to the lighter side, the two pans of the balance will come into equilibrium. Let us call the equilibrium the effect. What can we say about the causes?

Clearly, the one-pound weight added last was the temporally proximate cause of reaching an equilibrium. It was the event that immediately preceded the effect.[3] But its effectiveness depended on the presence of the other 99 pounds. These comprised the remote causes. All the weights had to be put in the pan to achieve the effect, and the temporal order in which they were placed there was not important. Regardless of the temporal order, there was one point at which the effect occurred, namely, when the last weight was added. Then the equilibrium was reached. Since the weights could be added in any order, if we ask, "What is *the* proximal cause of the equilibrium?" the answer would be, "The equality of weights on the two sides of the balance." When this has been reached, then nothing else can intervene. This, however, is only a tautology. We are saying that we have produced an equilibrium when we have achieved an equality of the two sides. But this is exactly the *definition* of equilibrium. In its logical sense the proximal cause is that which provides a definition. And the definition provides the necessity.

The concept of a definition is crucial in understanding *the* proximal cause and its relation to remote causes. For further analysis, let us suppose that we see three patients in a hospital, each with a broken leg. The first man, we learn, was struck by an automobile as he was crossing the street. The second had fallen while skiing. And the third was our friend with the metastatic carcinoma whose minor stumble had resulted in a fracture.

On further query we learn some of the remote causes for each case. The first man, on his way to getting a newspaper, was daydreaming, paid no attention to a traffic light, and did not see an oncoming car that had the right of way. Lots of people get newspapers, daydream while walking, and walk against the light, and yet suffer no harmful consequences.

The man who broke his leg while skiing was a beginner.

Moreover, he had a hangover from a party the night before and his reflexes were not reacting well. And he was trying to impress a girl-friend. All these individual factors occur frequently. None of them necessarily leads to a broken leg. Nevertheless, in this case the conjunction of remote causes did lead to the fracture.

The third case is similar. The man had been a heavy smoker for thirty years. He had paid no special attention to a persistent cough that had bothered him for several years, nor to a pain in the leg that he had noted a few months previously. Here again an array of remote causes culminated in the broken leg. And again we realize the lack of necessity for any one of them.

How did it happen that diverse remote causes, in different individuals, produced the same phenomenon, a fracture? It is no longer responsive to say, this man was struck by an automobile, that one fell on a ski slope, or that other one had a cancer. All the cases had something in common. What? The answer we seek would go something like this: in all cases the fracture occurred at the exact instant when the external force applied to the bone exceeded the cohesive strength of the bone substance. That was the exact moment when a cause transformed into an effect. There was an absolute necessity about it. Once the applied force exceeded the cohesive strength, no additional circumstance could exert any influence. This was the moment when *the* proximal cause was operative. And the same proximal cause occurs in every case of fracture, regardless of the attendant circumstances (i.e., of remote causes).

Proximal cause is thus completely different from any of the remote causes. It differs not only in temporal relationships but through its intrinsic logical nature. *The* proximal cause, in the sense used here, is precisely what we mean by the *definition* of the phenomenon under study. We define fracture to be the state in which the applied force exceeds the cohesive strength. When that occurs, we have a fracture, and we cannot avoid it, any more than a triangle can avoid having three sides. The necessity arises from the force of definition and thus constitutes a logical requirement.

Logicians, as well as scientists, have devoted a great deal of attention to the necessity that inheres in certain causal relationships. In any causal relation we find necessity when (and only when) the following conditions are met: "If A, then B, *and* if B, then A." The two conditions must both be satisfied. This is readily seen with the definition of fracture. If the applied force exceeds the cohesive force, then we have a fracture (if A, then B). If we have a fracture, then the applied force exceeded the cohesive strength (if B, then A). This formulation obviously does not apply to being struck by an automobile or to falling on a ski slope.

At this point the reader may demur. With a balance, we may put equal weights in the two pans and yet they may not come to an equilibrium; or, conversely, we may have an equilibrium, add more weight to one side, such as 0.01 milligram, and yet the equilibrium need not necessarily be disturbed. The scientist does not say that the definition was wrong, but only that other factors were operating that he had not yet taken into account. These factors would be additional remote causes that had escaped his attention. Thus, he may find that the fulcrum was not equidistant between the two pans; or perhaps the friction between the beam and the fulcrum was too great; or perhaps an unsuspected source of heat was producing a convection current that was acting on one of the pans. These would be unexpected intervening factors that interfered with the proximal cause. We might draw a comparison with the baseball game, wherein the runner, after hitting the ball over the fence, dropped dead before he touched home plate.

A definition must take into account the possible influence of many remote causes, and, in a sense, the more that a scientist can discover about remote causes, the more accurate will be his final definition. Here we encounter another important distinction, that between the actual and the ideal. Balances differ widely in precision and sensitivity, yet, no matter how sensitive the balance or how carefully shielded from environmental influences, there is always a limit to the precision and sensitivity. We cannot eliminate friction and inertia. An absolute equilibrium achieved through the addition of weights is an ideal. It constitutes a limiting condition that may be approached more and more closely by any actual balance, but as an idealized state can never be fully realized in the empirical world. The geometer can define a straight line, but in nature we can never find a line that is absolutely straight nor can we ever draw one, even though we can always approach more and more closely. In the world of nature a straight line, like a balance in equilibrium, represents a limiting condition. For practical purposes, however, the deviation from the ideal limit may make no difference.

We can see another difference between the example of the broken leg and the example of the balance. The broken leg is a yes-or-no state. You have it or you do not. It is not a limiting condition that might be approached asymptotically but never fully reached. An example even more striking than a fracture would be death. At any moment an organism is either dead or alive. The two are mutually exclusive and there is no intermediate zone, no question of "good enough for practical purposes" or "for the purposes of this context," as would obtain with the definition of equilibrium. We need the criteria for a yes-or-no answer. To cast light on this problem let us examine the cause of death.

## III

I will begin my comments with a moment of autobiography. In 1929, when I was a second-year medical student studying pathology, I attended an autopsy on a young child who had a massive lung abscess. The resident in pathology, performing the autopsy, demonstrated the findings and discussed them with the students. I remember asking the question, "Why did the child die?" The resident, with a biting scorn in his voice that I still remember, replied, "How would you expect her to live with an abscess like that?" The answer, of course, was entirely non-responsive to the question, but as a timid student in awe of an experienced resident, I did not press the point. Later, in a flash of *esprit d'escalier*, I thought of what I should have said:

"But she was alive yesterday and the abscess was just as big then."

Well, why *did* she die? Only much later did I appreciate the brutal truth, that the resident was too ignorant and too unsure of himself to say, "I don't know." The cause of death is perhaps the most difficult problem in biological science, and one for which there is as yet no good answer.

Yet every physician is expected to know the cause of death in any patient who dies under his care, and he must demonstrate this knowledge by filling out a death certificate. An autopsy may provide important information. The death certificate has no concern with what I call the proximal cause that applies to all dead people and is characterized by universality and necessity. The death certificate wants only a remote cause that has neither universality nor necessity. The answers are expected to be the names of individual diseases—lobar pneumonia, periarteritis nodosa, tuberculous meningitis, cerebral hemorrhage. Unacceptable would be an answer, "his heart stopped beating." The certificate wants to find out not why every patient died but why *this* patient died. Wanted is not the proximal cause but a suitable remote cause.

By their nature remote causes exert no necessity. Every case of lobar pneumonia does not lead to death, any more than every automobile accident leads to a broken leg. The certificate does not want any light on the question: why this patient with lobar pneumonia died while that one, with the same disease, did not. An infinite number of remote causes could bear on the event.

In this connection we recall the work of Rudolph Virchow, who in 1848 went to Upper Silesia to investigate the causes of typhus fever, then raging in epidemic form. In his report Virchow pointed not only to medical details but to various sociological factors, such as poverty, malnutrition, and crowding, as having causal significance. These would be remote causes, somewhat more remote than the actual infection, which in turn is more remote than *the* proximal cause of death.

The death certificate serves a purely practical function with two major components. One is medico-legal. A licensed physician, filling out the certificate, testifies that the patient did in fact die and that death resulted from "natural causes" rather than from some human agency, whether of crime or accident. Then, the death certificate is a means of gathering statistics, however dubious their validity. What is wanted is the name of a disease, and this name, once given, is arbitrarily called the cause, or sometimes the principal cause. The certificate also wants additional remote causes, through the questions "Due to?"

The proximal cause applies to all instances of a phenomenon and therefore has no differential value in distinguishing kinds, or sub-categories, or species. In regard to the cause of death, let us look at the popular answer, "The heart stopped beating." We know that actually this is not the proximal cause at all, but merely one remote cause, more proximal than many others but still far from *the* cause. With modern technology it is possible to keep a patient alive with no heart at all. The heart-beat is essential not for life but only for the unaided circulation of the blood. Suitable apparatus can provide a circulation in the total absence of either heart-beat or respiration.

As we get closer to *the* cause of death, we find that the circulation of the blood is not as essential as the presence of oxygen. But, again, it is not the mere presence of oxygen but its actual utilization within the cells. This utilization, however, is only one step in the activity of intracellular chemical reactions. And this is the area wherein our answer seems to lie, that highly specialized area of intracellular chemical reactions, whose details are the subject of sophisticated ongoing research.

Those of us who are not biochemists might be content to say that the proximal cause of death is the cessation of not-yet-understood chemical reactions within cells. But this is far from the whole story. In health many cells are constantly dying, and they are constantly being replaced. Some cell death is indeed requisite for health. Since the death of an individual person is quite distinct from the death of component cells, we must turn away from isolated cells to organs. But here we must specify "vital" organs. We know empirically that certain organs (such as placenta or spleen) can die within the body and yet the individual remains alive. But when we specify "vital" organs we are begging the question, for the term means "necessary for life," and that is precisely the point we are trying to investigate.

We must be alert to another example of begging the question. Historically, death has been popularly equated with cessation of the heart-beat. But since the heart may stop beating and then start in again, we insert the words "permanent" or "irreversible." But the word "irreversible" already implies the presence of death, and it is the conditions under which this takes place that we are trying to discover.

More recently attention has focussed on so-called brain death, the state where the cells of the brain have died (considered to have occurred when no function can be detected through electrical recordings) but other organs of the body still remain alive. Brain death merely emphasizes the accepted fact that different organs will die at different times. After the heart has (permanently) stopped beating, many other cell types can continue living for a while.

Granted that cells and organs die at different rates, we then face the problem: when does the individual-as-a-whole, the *person*, die? In addition to posing a logical problem, this question has legal and ethical significance, and is a sociological and philosophical problem in its own right.

Death, however, while it occurs gradually over a time span, has an unquestioned end-point. Chemical reactions go on at all times within the body. After death the character of these reactions, which we call "post-mortem change," is very different from the changes while the body is alive. Scientists try to identify the features that distinguish the one from the other. When they have succeeded in doing so, they will have discovered the proximal cause of death.

Meanwhile, when we try to identify the causes of death we must be content to deal with remote causes. These get closer and closer to the effect—death—until at some point we reach *the* proximal cause. Until we have reached this point, the course of events is, at least in theory, reversible. Something may intervene, and that something would be another remote cause. But, when the proximal cause is reached, it is no longer logically possible to intercalate any further remote cause. The process is irreversible. That is the point where Humpty-Dumpty falls, and then nothing can put him together again.

## IV

The examples used hitherto have in common some ready modes of discrimination that leave little doubt whether or not we are dealing with an example of the class under study. In ordinary circumstances we know that a leg is broken, that a balance is in equilibrium, or that a patient is dead. But if now, in our study of causation, we turn to a disease such as tuberculosis, we find a quite different situation. If we seek *the* cause of tuberculosis, our first problem is to identify individuals to whom we apply the diagnosis. Does he have tuberculosis? But to tell whether a given patient does in fact have tuberculosis may be quite difficult. Before we can hunt for the proximal cause of tuberculosis we must have a population of tuberculous patients and these might not be easy to identify. In Chapter 2 we have a historical sketch of the disease that can serve as a background for further analysis.

Consumption, we have seen, represented a pattern originally identified by a triad of symptoms—emaciation, cough, and hectic fever. These features seemed adequate to define typical cases of the class, but further study showed that the class was not at all precise, and that many other factors had to be taken into account.

When we regard the history of tuberculosis, we see in retrospect that research proceeded along three lines. Physicians had to define the condition more and more strictly. At the same time they studied the factors that seemed to have some role in inducing the disease (the remote causes). And they also tried to find the necessary cause, or the proximal cause, of the disease. Scientists investigate attendant circumstances, hoping that after sufficient study of these remote causes there will emerge the factors that all cases had in common—i.e., the proximal cause, with its necessity.

The early investigators recognized the relevance of the anatomical tubercle and its importance as a causal factor. The term
"acrid" provided a useful, even if hypothetical, agent. If an
exudation into the lung contained an acrid, there was potential
trouble. William Cullen declared: "The acrimony which discovers itself in the ulcers, existed before and produced the tubercles
themselves; *and it is to this acrimony that we must trace up the
cause of the phthisis following these tubercles.* This acrimony is
probably, in different cases, of different kinds; and it will not
be easy to determine its varieties." The prophecy is well worth
keeping in mind.[4] Other causal factors regarded as precursors
of phthisis included such clinical conditions as catarrh, scrofula,
and hemoptysis. These, as antecedent conditions that might or
might not be followed by phthisis, were remote causes of
phthisis. They were part of the total causal nexus but only in the
sense of remote causes.

In Chapter 2, I discussed the work of Bayle and of Laennec,
who made empirical correlations between clinical and anatomical
findings, and with increased insight greatly sharpened the definition of phthisis. Its essence lay in a progressive "disorganization" of the lung tissue, a concept that rendered the class of
phthisis patients more homogeneous.

By the 1830s microscopy introduced new observations, leading to new theories, but these raised stubborn problems. The
theory of the blastema illustrates the difficulties. If the anatomical tubercle was a major feature of the disease, any causal explanation had to tell how the tubercle arose. If the blastema
theory was correct, then the tubercles arose from a matrix-like
fluid that exuded from the blood. Investigators would then need
to trace causal links connecting the blood with the clinical manifestations. On the other hand, if the blastema theory was wrong
and the tubercle arose from pre-existing tissue elements, then
research would pursue a quite different set of causes.

There was the further problem of specificity. When Virchow
claimed that the features found in the tubercle could also be
found in diseases other than phthisis, he dealt a heavy blow to
the notion of specificity. And if we cannot point to anything

specific, how can we be sure what we are dealing with? And if we cannot be sure of that, how can we hunt for causes? Without a good circumscription of the disease entity, without a homogeneous group, we cannot achieve any precision in identifying causes. Only in a well-defined entity can we find some factor or factors that might be called the proximal cause. Remote causes are readily found, but remote causes, non-specific, can have more than one outcome. The proximal cause, on the other hand, will necessarily lead to one result—i.e., merge into it.

We thus see two sets of problems that in essence are related. First, what *is* the disease tuberculosis? How do you identify patients who suffer from it? And, second, once we have such a circumscription, what factors will *necessarily* bring it about? What is its proximal cause?

The solution to the first problem resulted from the work of Villemin and Koch, described in Chapter 2. Villemin showed the contagious nature of tuberculosis and Koch demonstrated the specific organism. He thereby added a crucial limiting condition to the causal network. None of the remote causes would lead to tuberculosis unless the specific tubercle bacillus were present. This discovery allowed physicians to speak with complete confidence about the disease entity. They could say with assurance, "This patient has tuberculosis." The presence of the bacillus seemed to provide a sharp criterion. Physicians could point to various causal factors, all of which, with one exception, might be shared with other diseases. The exception was the tubercle bacillus, found only in tuberculosis.

This criterion, however, had negative value only and did not involve any causal necessity. If the patient did not harbor the bacillus, he did not have tuberculosis; but if the bacillus was present in his body, he did not necessarily have the disease. The bacillus was not the proximal cause. Other factors were needed that we can lump together under the term "susceptibility." This condenses into a single word many extremely complex immunological properties. We can speak, tautologically but usefully, of defenses, without trying to specify their details.

Physicians have often regarded the bacillus as a "necessary but not sufficient cause." The older writers, who used Latin, had the term *causa sine qua non*, the causal factor without which the disease would not occur. To translate this as "necessary cause" carries distorting overtones: a better rendition would be "indispensable factor." Ordinarily more than a single indispensable factor is required for a definition.

According to present-day definitions, when the tubercle bacilli enter the lungs and grow and multiply, then the patient has pulmonary tuberculosis. If an active agent is multiplying, this means that any defense mechanism is inadequate.

In the 17th century Morton, trying to separate those patients who had phthisis from those who did not, offered a definition, but, as we have seen, this did not exert any necessity. We may properly ask, "Why not?" The answer, I suggest, relates to the difference between description and explanation. Morton, with his criteria of hectic fever, emaciation, and purulent sputum, was defining a class on the basis of what he directly observed. He gave an empirical descriptive account. This the older writers would regard as natural history. When, however, we try to explain the phenomena, we are concerned with natural philosophy, which penetrates to deeper levels and involves theory and inference rather than merely immediate observation. In contrast to description, which is empirical, explanation deals with causes and is rational. Science, the outgrowth of natural philosophy, seeks definitions based not on description but on explanation through causes. This is rational interpretation that the scientist tries to make completely rigorous.[5]

When we deal with causes, rigor inheres only in those identified as proximal. In more modern terms this means the factors that obey the formulations, "If A, then B; *and* if B, then A," where A is what we call the cause and B the effect. In our present example tuberculosis is the effect (B) while the proximate cause (A) is the conjunction of the indispensable factors. If the patient harbors the tubercle bacillus and lacks adequate defense mechanisms, we know that he has tuberculosis; and if he has tuberculosis, we know that he harbors the bacilli and has insufficient immunological defenses. This, as the proximal cause, provides a rigorous definition that conveys necessity.[6]

V

In distinguishing empirical from causal definitions we find an instructive example in the disease yellow fever. In 1881 Carlos Finlay had presented evidence that the disease was transmitted by the mosquito now called *Aedes aegypti*. The actual proof, however, came only from the brilliant and heroic work of Walter Reed and his associates at the turn of the century. They showed conclusively that this mosquito was the natural vector of the disease, and they worked out the specific details. They also showed that the infectious agent, transmitted by the mosquito after a suitable incubation period, was not a bacterium, as earlier investigators had wrongly thought, but an agent that could pass through a fine porcelain filter—a so-called filterable virus. However, the actual agent escaped isolation and identification.

After scientists learned the mode of transmission, they were able to control the spread of the disease. By warring on the mosquito they made fabulous progress in epidemiology, and virtually eliminated the disease in many areas where it had been endemic. Nevertheless the agent had not been identified.

In our terminology the mosquito was as much a causal factor as the unknown agent. And the breeding places of the mosquito were also part of the causal network, which ramified into aspects of climate, cultural habits, and the like. In the older terminology every aspect of this linkage would be a remote cause, but the proximal cause remained unknown.

In the second decade of the 20th century the microbiologist Hideyo Noguchi (1876-1928) sought the actual transmissible agent. Obviously, before he could undertake his studies he needed a population of patients who had the disease. He went to Ecuador, where yellow fever was still endemic, and there he was given access to 172 "typical" cases. From several of these patients he recovered a spirochete that he claimed fulfilled Koch's postulates regarding causation. The spirochete could pass through a filter, could be transmitted by *Aedes aegypti* after a suitable incubation, could be isolated in pure culture, reacted to antibodies in convalescent serum, and could reproduce in guinea pigs a disease similar to yellow fever in humans. By adducing evidence derived from pathology, microbiology, immunology, and epidemiology, Noguchi claimed that his spirochete was "the" cause of yellow fever.

There was, however, one serious flaw that he did not take into account. What assurance did he have that he was dealing with yellow fever? When other workers in different parts of the world could not confirm his findings, certain assumptions in his reasoning became evident. Noguchi assumed that the patients from whom he recovered the spirochete had yellow fever. He was relying on the clinical diagnosis made by experienced clinicians. And they, in turn, depended on diagnostic criteria that were purely empirical, defined in clinical and not in causal terms.

Eventually it turned out that the clinicians who had gathered together a group of "yellow-fever patients" had collected a composite group. Some were genuine yellow-fever patients; others were suffering from an ailment that had features in common with yellow fever but was an entirely distinct disease entity— spirochetal jaundice. It was from these latter patients that Noguchi had recovered a specific transmissible agent, but it was the agent for spirochetal jaundice (now called leptospirosis) and not yellow fever.

After Noguchi had recovered spirochetes from patients whom he thought had yellow fever, he boldly proclaimed that the spirochete was "the" causative agent in yellow fever. Other scientists, however, working with "real" yellow fever, could not confirm his findings, indicated that his evidence was flimsy, and denied his assertions. The tragic aftermath is well known. Noguchi, having his own doubts, was incapable of acknowledging his own errors. To pursue further studies on cases whose clinical identification as yellow fever would not be questioned, he went to Africa, and there he succumbed to the disease he was investigating.[7]

Today the rigorous diagnosis of yellow fever depends on the isolation and identification of the virus or the demonstration of the specific antibodies. Technically these procedures are far more difficult than is the case with the identification of the tubercle bacillus. But the criteria, although more difficult to meet, have the same logical force that we have in the more familiar tuberculosis, and the concept of proximal cause is strictly comparable.

## VI

Much of the confusion attending the term "cause" rests on the failure to distinguish between *a* cause and *the* cause, between a singular event and a generalization. *The* cause is meaningful under two conditions, one of which represents history, the other science, where history deals with the particular event and science with classes and generalizations.

For the unique event the cause is the totality of factors that led to it. As Mandelbaum says, "The cause of an effect is simply the process that terminates in the effect: the cause is the whole set of actual ongoing occurrences or events that resulted in this, and no other particular event."[8] Such a view agrees with the statement of Riverius, quoted above (p. 206). If in a particular event *the* cause is the totality of factors that led to it, then each of the separate factors would be a remote cause so that the entire conjunction terminated in the event called the effect. Of course, some factors, some threads in the causal network, are more remote than others.

The older physicians gave specific qualifying names to the various factors, such as *causa sine qua non*, procatarctic cause, continuing cause, and the like. Any of these, *without qualification*, would be *a* cause; when the qualification is used, the particle *the* is appropriate. Unfortunately, modern writers wanted to use the word *the* and at the same time eliminate the qualifying term. They spoke of *the* cause when they meant some remote cause that seemed especially relevant to the interests of the inquirer. A psychoanalyst, for example, would have one set of interests, an insurance adjuster quite a different set. But for any singular event *the* cause is the totality of antecedent factors or the sum of the remote causes.

Since we cannot meaningfully envision a totality, we necessarily abstract and isolate. In the process we apply the term *the* to what we consider especially important, while everything else is downgraded in one or another terminology. "Causal condition" is a popular term.[9] There is no objection to this as a matter of convenience, provided we recognize its basic inadequacy.

The situation is quite different when we deal with generalizations or "laws" of science, and here we deal with the second of our major groupings. Science, in contrast to history, pays no heed to the infinite richness of the particular. Science artificially isolates certain observed sequences and tries to find the conditions under which they *do* occur and the conditions under which they *must* occur. To achieve this, the earlier physicians and philosophers sought the proximal cause, as the acme of investigation. I suggest the similarities of this point of view to the Aristotelian concept of definition, which sought the "essence" of a thing.

*TREATMENT*

——————◁▷◁▷——————

## CHAPTER 11

# Reflections on Blood-Letting

*Today doctors can* do *something for their patients.* Of course, the older physicians prescribed vast quantities of drugs and performed various therapeutic indignities like bleeding and sweating, but—so runs a popular mythology—in the old days treatment led chiefly to disaster—unless the healing power of nature cured the patients in spite of the physicians.

Blood-letting has become a symbol for whatever was bad in earlier medical practice. Everyone seems to know that George Washington died from excessive blood-lettings when he lay ill with a sore throat; and that Benjamin Rush, with fanatic intensity, almost exsanguinated his patients under the guise of helping them. Today, on the other hand, we have a constant succession of new wonder-drugs and other near-miraculous treatments that are *really* effective. And anyone (like myself) who remains somewhat skeptical quickly gets referred to mortality statistics and to the decline in the overall death rate.

Yet blood-letting should not be condemned unheard. Why did it become popular? How did the physicians explain its apparent success? How and why did it get superseded? If we answer these questions in regard to blood-letting, we will find surprising similarities to modern medical practice and perceive some important linkages between past and present.

No one knows the origin of blood-letting as a mode of therapy. Apparently the ancient Egyptians practiced it at least as long ago as 2500 B.C. For our purposes we need go no farther back than Hippocrates. He used blood-letting "to get rid of redundant matter in the system"; to redistribute the blood, or, in the technical vocabulary of the time, to change "the deter-

mination of the blood to or from particular parts"; and to restore
a free movement of the blood and animal spirits in cases where
they were supposed to be stagnant or obstructed. Blood-letting
was especially indicated in violent inflammation—pleurisy,
quinsy (the disease from which George Washington suffered),
and inflammation of the lung. Hippocrates also recommended
bleeding to alleviate difficulty in breathing and to relieve pain.
In fevers he would let blood only if the febrile state was connected with some "topical inflammation"—i.e., was a "symptomatic" rather than a "primary" fever.

Henry Clutterbuck (1767-1856), writing in 1839, noted that
these recommendations were "unaided, for the most part, by the
lights of anatomy, physiology, or the other auxiliary sciences";
and he commented, "how little . . . has been added to the stock
of real practical knowledge since his time."[1]

Here we have a concept of immense importance. Hippocrates
was entirely ignorant of the theories of later science. Nevertheless, his therapeutic advice, his actual medical practice, was
comparable to that employed in the early 19th century. His
precepts had stood the test of time and had not been outmoded
by theoretical advances. Clutterbuck regarded therapeutics as a
matter of practical experience. The validity of blood-letting
rested on observation and experience.

I suggest that venesection originally became established as a
major therapeutic agent *because it worked*—at least, often enough
to induce confidence in its effectiveness. I have often been asked
whether blood-letting had any value or whether it was a mere
superstition that ignorance had fastened on the general public.
My questioners usually express surprise when I insist that in
many conditions venesection had great value, even according to
modern concepts.

For example, if a person with high-blood pressure and a severe headache should have a spontaneous nosebleed, he would
feel better. The improvement might be only temporary, but the
relief would unquestionably be associated with the loss of blood.
In lobar pneumonia a large part of the lung gets filled with
exudate so that the amount of functioning pulmonary tissue is

sharply reduced. The heart has to pump the same volume of blood through a diminished capillary bed in the lungs. Under certain conditions this can produce congestion in the normal parts of the lung. Reducing the blood volume through venesection can give considerable relief, again on a temporary basis.

Vascular congestion in the lungs can place a burden on the right side of the heart. Any disproportion between the volume of blood and the ability of the heart to pump it may improve after venesection. So too with the difficulty in breathing that for Hippocrates served as one indication for blood-letting. Today we fully recognize that many conditions can benefit from a reduction of the total volume of circulating fluid. We have various ways today of accomplishing the end in view, but, before improved methods were known, physicians had to rely on the available modes of therapy, and blood-letting was especially important.

II

*Eighteenth-Century Views*

Historically, the major indications for blood-letting have been the relief of inflammation and the treatment of fevers, conditions that in the aggregate comprised a large part of medical practice. The case for blood-letting rested on two grounds. One was its practical value. That venesection did in fact help in certain conditions was a matter of experience. The second support lay in conformity to theory. Medical doctrine could give a well-articulated explanation as to why and how blood-letting worked. To be sure, the theory changed from time to time and reasons once accepted might be discarded later. Nevertheless, blood-letting could never be called a blind empiricism. It had a rationale.

To perceive a unity of development we need go no farther back than the teachings of Boerhaave (1668-1738). For him inflammation resulted principally from a mechanical obstruction of vessels. The obstruction might derive from a contraction of the vessels, an impaction of particles (such as red blood cells), or a thickening—"spissitude"—of the blood. The obstruction produced the characteristic marks of inflammation: swelling, redness, heat, and pain.[2]

Any vascular obstruction was made worse by the force of the heartbeat, which, acting from behind, drove the impacted blood cells deeper into the small vessels and thus intensified the inflammation. One way of resolving an inflammation was to relieve the impacting force resulting from the arterial pressure. This the physician could accomplish by "diminishing the force of the arterial blood by bleeding and purging." When this forward pressure was relieved, the "action of the vessels" could "overcome" the obstructing material. "So soon therefore as the quantity and impetus of the distending blood has been diminished by bleeding and purging," then other remedies could act as a "gentle stimulus" to the vascular fibers, so that these might "break or divide the obstructing particles" and thus permit them to pass through the ends of the vessels.[3]

Especially to be noted is this "action" of the small vessels. For Boerhaave the vessels performed the functional activities that today we assign to cells. The reader should appreciate the rough analogy between "vessels" in the older terminology and "cells" in the modern.[4]

Inflammation, resulting from obstruction of vessels for whatever reason, had a close relationship to fevers. In fever there was not a total obstruction but rather an impediment, for which some change in the blood was a major factor. The essence of fever was deemed to lie not, as today, in an increased body temperature, but in a rapid pulse. This rapid pulse in turn reflected the activity of the heart. For Boerhaave the rapid pulse represented an increased "action" of the heart. Diminishing the quantity of the blood would weaken the motion of the circulation. "We may reduce the force of the fever to a just moderation, in proportion to the quantity of blood which is drawn." Bleeding abates the violence of a fever because it abates the "action" of the heart.[5]

William Cullen (1710-1790) succeeded Boerhaave as the leading clinician and theorist of the century. He rejected the concept of a thickening of the blood as a factor in either fever or inflammation and similarly rejected the notion that obstruction was a stoppage of the vessels. All the available evidence, he thought, argued against such a concept. Instead he invoked an *"increased action of the vessels"* that manifests itself as a spasm of the vascular channels; this spasm prevents the vessels from transmitting the blood brought to them.[6]

The difference between Boerhaave and Cullen shows a considerable shift in thinking. Instead of a mechanical blockage from an impaction of cells, Cullen invoked a functional obstruction or hindrance resulting from spasm. This marked a change from a mechanical to a dynamic interpretation, with greater emphasis on physiology. Cullen agreed that in inflammation the passage of blood through the vessels was hindered, but the reason lay in the spasm or "increased action" of the vessels. A great many remote causes might trigger this increased action. Some substances could irritate by their "acrimony"; or trauma or heat or cold or some comparable agent might act; or there might be merely "an increased impetus of the blood determined to a particular part"—a statement that, if regarded critically, means that no remote cause was identified.[7]

To cure an inflammation the physician might neutralize or correct any acrids, or he might remove the spasm of the involved part. This he could accomplish "by remedies applied either to the whole system, or to the part itself." The overall idea was "that a spasm of the extreme vessels, however induced, proves an irritation to the heart and arteries; and that this continues till the spasm is relaxed or overcome." To accomplish this the physician should try to "moderate the violence of the reaction." He must "diminish the action" of the heart and arteries. If we diminish the quantity of fluid, we will "diminish the activity of the sanguiferous system" and relieve the spasm. This is accomplished most readily by blood-letting and purging.[8]

Cullen recommended caution in blood-letting, for its use "requires much discernment and skill." Many factors must be taken into account—among others the nature of the disease, its causes, the amount of "phlogistic diathesis" present, the age, strength, and vigor of the patient, and the appearance of the blood as it issues from the body. He also emphasized means other than blood-letting for removing the spasm, such as anti-spasmodics and diluents.[9]

Although Cullen's concepts of physiology and physiopathology differed from those of Boerhaave, the therapeutic agents were in essence similar. When should the practitioner use vigorous remedies such as venesection and purging, and when milder remedies? Here the judgment of the physician was of critical importance. When fevers were primarily inflammatory, with a strong reaction of the system, strong measures were needed to "reduce" the vigor of that reaction. On the other hand, some fevers were characterized by weakness and prostration, and should not be treated by venesection. The physician had to rely on general indications.

Of special importance in the history of blood-letting is John Brown (1735-1788), a pupil of Cullen, who propounded an original system that for a while had a considerable vogue. Brown grounded his doctrine on a fundamental principle that he called "excitability," a basic property of living matter. We can think of this as the *capacity to react*. The correlative principle was *excitement*, representing the stimuli, either external or internal, that acted on the body. Too much excitement was bad, constituting what he called the "sthenic" diseases. Too little excitement was equally bad, inducing *asthenic* diseases, characterized by debility. A sthenic disease might overstimulate, exhaust the excitability, and thus lead to an indirect debility.[10]

The role of the physician was clear. Within certain limits he treated by opposites—diminish the excitement if excessive, increase it if insufficient. To diminish the excitement in sthenic diseases, blood-letting was especially important. However, over-treatment was bad, for it might change a disease into its opposite. Too great depletion might bring the patient into indirect debility.

In Brown's writings we find a reckless use of terms, little objectivity, and no firm criteria. If excessive stimuli, through "indirect debility," could induce a clinical picture indistinguishable from deficient stimuli, a student might excusably be puzzled. In Brown's concepts, if the patient did not do well the physician had probably stimulated when he should have depleted, and vice versa, but it was very difficult to tell ahead of time.

Brown had apparently simplified the practice of medicine, but actually he had obscured the need for careful discrimination and for the nice judgment on which Cullen had insisted. Brown's doctrine made it quite easy to go to great excesses in blood-letting. If in the opinion of the physician the patient suffered from too much excitement, the therapy was simple—diminish the excitement through blood-letting. The dangers of such an approach are seen in Benjamin Rush (1745-1813), who pursued a career of frenetic blood-letting. He was a conscientious physician and a man of great intellectual attainments, but abysmally deficient in critical attitude. Although he denied dependence on Brown, Rush manifestly relied on the same basic concepts and failed to take any part in the gradual progress toward objectivity that was making itself felt by the end of the 18th century.[11]

### III

The first third of the 19th century, for all of its advances in the basic sciences, did not bring about any significant changes in therapy. If anything, under the influence of Broussais in France and Benjamin Rush in this country, the trend toward voluminous blood-letting increased. The moderation and careful judgment that Cullen had recommended were too often replaced by a reckless abandon. Although the basic sciences were making excellent progress, they did not influence practice until the second half of the century.

In the first forty years or so of the 19th century the practitioners had to rely, for the most part, on traditional wisdom. The teachers who dominated this period spread doctrines that they themselves had acquired in an earlier tradition. The new advances were being made chiefly by younger men. For significant changes to take place in practice, a new generation first had to be trained in the new methods, the new spirit. Only when these men, with their newer learning, reached a dominant position in medical education could the older tradition be subdued. In regard to blood-letting we see this happening around the middle of the century.

To examine the status of blood-letting at the end of the 1830s we will turn again to Clutterbuck. He had long advocated moderate and judicious blood-letting, noting that this was one of the most effective medicinal agents, "powerful for good or for evil, according to the judgment and discrimination with which it is administered." All too often, he admitted, it was abused, and only careful observation of its effects could indicate its real value. This, he admitted, was only an empirical judgment. Since we have insufficient knowledge of basic causes, we must rely on "observation and experience, as the only guides." He was saying, in effect: "We do not know how blood-letting works, nor why it works in some cases and not in others." He was convinced, however, that it *did* work, even though he admitted that in many cases where blood-letting was effective (e.g., apoplexy and violent inflammation) the patients might recover without using this remedy.

We do not need to follow the intricacies of his discussion, but can go directly to his conclusion. Blood-letting is effective in "a great variety of morbid states that differ widely from one another." It is a "soveriegn remedy" in a wide range of inflammatory conditions. It is an antispasmodic. It relieves pain. It sometimes promotes and sometimes restrains the "natural discharges."

Clutterbuck offered a hypothesis to explain these observations: "The most intelligible explanation of the matter appears to be this: that by any considerable loss of blood, however occasioned, all vital movements, morbid as well as healthy, are more or less disturbed. In this respect, therefore, blood-letting resembles, in its effect, other sudden and powerful impressions of the system." Cold baths, extreme pain, terror, can all produce a similar "commotion in the system." So too with blood-letting. Its value lies in the "impression on the system" that it makes.

The intensity of this impression will depend on a number of factors.[12]

This type of explanation has an 18th-century stamp. It differs markedly from what we like to think of as 19th-century thought—the careful analytical procedures followed by research men like Liebig, or Magendie, or Claude Bernard. Clutterbuck could not offer any precise or detailed explanation, but he did not feel the need for such precision. He rested primarily on the irrefutable "fact" that blood-letting *did* help, even though theory could not tell him why.

A comparable point of view we find in James Wardrop (1782-1869), a leading London surgeon of that era, who in the late 1830s published a book on the curative effects of blood-letting.[13] For Wardrop blood-letting served two principal aims—to diminish the "action of the heart and arteries in inflammatory diseases" and to remove an excess of fluid (or plethora). The blood-letting could be either general or local. The general procedure—venesection—he recommended for "a febrile disturbance throughout the system." The evidence for such a constitutional disturbance lay not in the mere frequency of the pulse but in its quality. The physician must identify an "incompressibility"—i.e., a difficulty in obliterating the pulse by simple digital pressure. (Today we tend to correlate this property with the blood pressure, but Wardrop had no means of taking the blood pressure.) Incompressibility was a crucial sign that always called for venesection, but other signs, such as a firm or full or wiry pulse, might also indicate the propriety.

Wardrop recommended allowing the blood to flow until the patient fainted, by which time the force of the pulse would diminish. If after many hours the pulse started to "rise" again, the bleeding should be repeated "until the strength of the heart and arteries be again subdued."

In local inflammation, where there was no general disturbance of the system, he recommended leeches rather than venesection. He also mentioned special instances of removing blood from the actual site of the inflammation, including cases of "blood poisoning" and "phlegmon." In one particular case that he described, an extensive inflammation of the hand and arm arose "from a poisoned wound of the finger, received when opening a putrid body." The patient had already been copiously bled, until the pulse had "sunk," but the swelling and pain persisted. The surgeon then secured good results by "making deep and extensive incisions" through the area of inflammation. "Several pounds of blood" were discharged through the incision, and the patient made an excellent recovery. The good results Wardrop attributed entirely "to the profuse bleeding which generally follows the incisions." He gave details of several similar cases.

Actually, Wardrop was recommending the operation of incision and drainage, highly appropriate in certain cases of infection. Today, the important feature is adequate drainage. Wardrop knew nothing of streptococcus infection. The good results from incision and drainage he attributed to the loss of blood during the operation, i.e., to local blood-letting. The patient's recovery strengthened the belief that the therapeutic value lay in the blood loss.

Wardrop was highly discriminating in his indications for blood-letting. He fully realized that abstraction of blood might have bad consequences but that unchecked inflammation might have worse. The physician must not bleed indiscriminately but must use his skill to determine when blood should be let and to what extent. One case that Wardrop cites indicates some of the difficulties.

In an accident a man suffered an extremely severe trauma to the knee. Wardrop first saw him twenty-four hours after the accident, when the knee was swollen, tense, and painful. The man seemed not to have recovered from the initial shock, for his skin was cold and his pulse low. There was no "febrile excitement." However, ten hours later the pulse, although not increased in frequency, "had a contracted feel—there was a difficulty in compressing it." This Wardrop interpreted as a warning of approaching inflammation, and he bled the patient copiously "until the pulse should be quite subdued." He felt that "the most energetic means" must be taken "to prevent the access of inflammation," for otherwise the patient might lose the limb or even his life.

The patient lost seventy-four ounces of blood "before the pulse faded." He remained for four days in a "state of prostration, and with the vigour of the organs of circulation quite subdued." Then he slowly recovered and "in three or four weeks the prostration caused by the blood-letting . . . were completely overcome" and he also gradually recovered from the local effects of the severe trauma.[13]

In retrospect we see the handicaps under which Wardrop labored. He knew nothing about specific bacteria and, since he wrote before the advent of cell theory, he had no notion of the microscopic changes in the various kinds of inflammation. He could not distinguish inflammation that accompanied infection from that which attended severe but aseptic trauma. He was unable to make any meaningful correlations between body reactions and causal agents. Furthermore, inflammation was only in part a local reaction. For him it might also be a reaction of the whole body, identified by the character of the pulse.

The situation changed, but only gradually. The decade of the 1840s showed a great upsurge of enthusiasm among the younger men, who embraced new ideas and challenged the proponents of the old. The disputes about blood-letting illustrate the differences between the old and the new, and show the merits and drawbacks attending each side of the controversy. One such conflict came to a head in Edinburgh in the early 1850s.

## IV

In the mid 1850s there occurred in Edinburgh an episode that shows how problems related to blood-letting may ramify in unexpected ways. When we unravel the arguments, we see that the differences can be reduced to a few disagreements that we can sharply pinpoint. And, as so often happens in arguments, when the issues are finally clarified, we find that the disputants were not talking about the same things. Hence both could be right, each within his own frame of reference, and each could be wrong when placed in his opponent's perspective.

The conflict involved the old and the new. A tradition once dominant and respected found itself challenged by newer ideas propounded by younger men who, in the enthusiasm of youth and the pride of their "modern" science, trampled upon views that had served well for generations.

In the second half of the 18th century Edinburgh had become the outstanding medical center in the entire world. After the death of Boerhaave, the leadership had passed from Leiden to Edinburgh, where William Cullen, with whose views we have already become acquainted, was the most prominent physician. Among the other leaders, although of lesser stature, were John Gregory (1724-1772) and James Gregory (1753-1821). By the middle of the 19th century this glory had already faded and the primacy in medicine had shifted first to Paris and then to Berlin. Edinburgh, although still important as a medical center, was basking quietly in its former eminence, even though no longer the world leader.

In the middle of the 19th century the leading physician in Edinburgh was William Pultney Alison (1790-1859), the grandson of John Gregory, the nephew of James Gregory, and the direct intellectual descendant of William Cullen. He typified the older generation and the older traditions.

John Hughes Bennett (1812-1875), whom we have already met in the story of tuberculosis, represented the younger generation. After receiving his medical degree from Edinburgh in 1837, he spent the next four years in post-graduate study in Paris and Berlin, immersing himself in the newest medical currents. He returned to Edinburgh to teach and to practice. Over the years he had become an accomplished microscopist. No longer satisfied with clinical observation alone, he realized the importance of pathology for understanding disease. He taught the medical students the doctrines prevalent in the advanced circles in Europe, doctrines that in many ways ran counter to the teachings of Cullen and Gregory.

In a lecture to the medical students Bennett condemned the practice of blood-letting in pneumonia, a practice that, as we have seen, had a long tradition in its favor and was still being supported by Alison. Bennett, although a native son, was a relative newcomer to the Edinburgh faculty and, moreover, had been trained largely in a foreign tradition. When he attacked the practices favored by Cullen, the Gregories, and Alison, he was in a way attacking the national pride of Scotland. He aroused intense resentment among the medical leaders, and the resulting conflict raged passionately. Today we have only the traces—the published papers, the discussions as reported in Society Transactions, and letters to the editor of the *Edinburgh Medical Journal*.[14] From these traces we can reconstruct the attitudes toward blood-letting in mid-century, and the reasons for the different views.

When we eliminate all the rhetoric, we can see clear points of agreement and equally clear points of difference. There was no dispute that the statistics on pneumonia showed a definite decline in mortality during the preceding half century. Furthermore, the practice of blood-letting was losing ground and was not being practiced as vigorously as heretofore. These would represent the agreed "facts." But what did they mean? The facts received quite different interpretations, and unravelling the differences provides considerable insight into some problems in the methods of science.

The discussion, we must always keep in mind, concerned the value of blood-letting in pneumonia. But what do we mean by pneumonia? Bennett regarded the condition in terms of underlying pathology—an inflammation that affected the air-sacs of the lung. As one of the leading microscopists of his time, he defined pneumonia in terms that he could perceive under the microscope. In pneumonia there was an exudation from the bloodstream into the lung tissues. This exudate filled the air spaces and coagulated but, if the course was favorable, would soften, liquefy, and eventually get absorbed back into the blood. Blood-letting, as a therapeutic procedure, could not affect the exudate nor alter the sequence of events as observed under the microscope. Hence blood-letting was not only useless in pneumonia but worse than useless, for it would only deplete the strength of the patient. The decline in mortality in pneumonia Bennett attributed to the lessened incidence of blood-letting in this disease.

Alison had no expertise in pathology. When he spoke of

pneumonia, he referred entirely to clinical experience. And clinically the cases that were being diagnosed as pneumonia were quite different in the mid-fifties from what they had been at the turn of the century. The old types of pneumonia that Cullen had described and for which blood-letting had been regarded as beneficial (i.e., in what we call lobar pneumonia) were no longer as prevalent as formerly. Instead, physicians were seeing new kinds of pneumonia—mild bronchopneumonia, in our terminology—with a quite different clinical course. For these new types, blood-letting was not beneficial. Alison pointed out—a matter of general agreement—that the new methods of diagnosis, such as auscultation and percussion, had altered the diagnosis of pulmonary disease. With these new methods the practitioner could detect exudation into the lung that was attended with little danger and formerly would have escaped notice.

In former times these cases would not have been called pneumonia. Now, however, with improved diagnosis, cases designated pneumonia gave rise to statistics that had no relevance to the cases that Cullen had seen. Alison thus placed his finger on an important pitfall in statistical reasoning: were the cases under consideration a homogeneous group? Pathologically they had features in common, namely, exudate in the alveoli, but clinically they were quite variable.

Alison did not use the term "clinical entity" but he clearly had in mind the equivalent concept. Pneumonia once had been considered a single disease, described by a single term. Whereas today we would say that this one term covers many clinical entities (as well as pathological entities), Alison said only that the disease was changing. He did not try to break down a single category into discrete sub-categories, for he had no criteria to go on. He merely emphasized that what was being *called* pneumonia was no longer what it had been. With our present knowledge of bacteriology, we can make all manner of discriminations not available to Alison. He could fall back only on vaguely conceived clinical data, for which there were no sharp defining features.

In regard to blood-letting the different points of view led to different conclusions. Bennett said, in effect, that blood-letting was never any good in pneumonia, but only now, with better methods of diagnosis and a sounder knowledge of pathology, could the lack of value be proved. Alison declared, in essence, that the available data had no bearing on the question as to whether blood-letting was effective *in the cases that Cullen had seen* (i.e., in what we call lobar pneumonia). The newer types of pneumonia, for which blood-letting had little benefit (i.e., bronchopneumonia), had nothing to do with the older cases for which blood-letting had been beneficial. Alison denied that knowledge derived from auscultation or microscopy could over-throw the clinical evidence that the older physicians—highly reliable observers—had adduced. The statistical evidence was not relevant.

Each of the disputants had his own impervious bias. For Ben-nett blood-letting was ineffectual in combatting inflammation, and anything that even suggested the contrary was manifestly wrong. Alison had his own immovable position: that blood-let-ting was clinically helpful in many cases of pneumonia. Any evidence that even implied the contrary was unacceptable. Nei-ther side could satisfactorily define the disease they were talking about.

The tide, however, was moving against Alison. For thought-ful physicians, reliance on experience alone, without a rationale, was not in keeping with scientific medicine. Advances in phys-iology, pathology, and chemistry more and more impaired the conceptual basis for blood-letting. Increased knowledge about inflammation and its many different kinds, and above all the discovery of bacteria as specific agents, all helped to discourage phlebotomy. Blood-letting underwent a steady decline in popu-larity in the last third of the 19th century.

Nevertheless, as Risse has convincingly shown, toward the end of the century there began a quiet renaissance in phlebotomy that had considerable vogue until the growth of chemotherapy in the mid-20th century. For the details of the movement and its limitation, Risse's paper is an excellent source. The trend, however, is tangential to our own story.[15]

V

From the history of blood-letting we can draw important lessons. First, the practice that began in pure empirical fashion accords with the soundest principles of medical science *in certain cases*. However, and this is the second lesson, what we now know was truly beneficial in some instances had been uncritically extended to other cases where it was of no value. Only relatively recent studies have been able to separate with assurance the cases where venesection was useless, or worse than useless, from those where it conferred provable benefit.

Third, even where it conferred real benefit (the cant way of saying this is, "scientifically verified") there were undesirable side-effects. Possible harmful side-effects are, of course, the great bugbear of all therapy, and the problem is even more pressing today than ever before. For example, the delayed sequellae of radiation, with disastrous results in some cases, is an obvious instance, and the whole concept of iatrogenic disease—where the remedy prescribed for one disease induces another disease—is quite vivid today.

Fourth, scientific progress can often eliminate the harmful side-effects while permitting the physician to reach the desired goal through other means. The great drawback in venesection was the loss of red cells. Modern science now permits the physician to restore the red cells to the patient. As a limiting case we can point to "exchange transfusions" as a form of blood-letting—drawing off the "bad humors" while avoiding the side-effects of the older procedure. Or again, the physician can now treat "plethora," not by venesection, but by controlling the sodium levels in the blood.

The history of blood-letting teaches us some methodological principles that apply equally well to the most sophisticated modern advances: blind adherence to a therapeutic regimen can cause trouble, and so can the uncritical extension of a remedy from one disease to another, and so can the failure to critically evaluate any clinical improvement in relation to the remedy. The important words here are "blind adherence," "uncritical extension," and "critically evaluate." The devotees of blood-letting sinned in all three respects.

We must, however, wonder to what extent our modern therapy is equally uncritical and to what degree present-day physicians prescribe (or otherwise treat) by rote. For example, if a physician prescribes antibiotics and the result is not all that he expected, a critic may say that if only the antibiotics had been given earlier, or in larger doses, or continued longer, the results would have been different. The possibility that the therapy was not appropriate for the condition that the patient actually had is an alternative that the physician might not readily accept. It is too easy to find reasons for an unfavorable result, reasons that *for the individual case* can never be gainsaid.

The proponents of blood-letting were quite prone to this type of reasoning. Thomas Sydenham, for example, reported a case where after blood-letting the patient was much improved. Sydenham recommended one further blood-letting, but the friends of the patient objected. "I explained to them that one more bleeding alone was wanting, and that that would place him out of danger. . . . In one word, I said that he must be bled or die." No more blood was let, and unfortunately the patient died. For Sydenham the death occurred for lack of one more blood-letting. It is easy to say in retrospect that he would have died anyway.[16]

I raise the question whether the same type of reasoning does not often occur today. Where a physician is convinced of the intrinsic value of the therapy, the failure to have a successful result in some individual case is always easy to explain away. If the patient recovers, the remedy gets the credit. If the patient does not recover, one explanation might be that the remedy was inappropriate. This, however, is not readily accepted. Far easier is the alternative explanation: that the remedy was appropriate but given in too small doses or not soon enough.

At the present time physicians hold to an ideal of rigorous controls, with double blind trials, to determine the "true" effectiveness. Yet this ideal of scientific method, admirable as a tool for establishing generalizations, may have little relevance for the individual case. A remedy that proved helpful in a high percentage of cases may or may not be effective in one particular patient.

Some of the difficulties attending the establishment of controls I will take up in Chapter 13, on Scientific Method. But in relation to the merits of blood-letting I would draw attention to a modern problem in therapeutics. In 1970 John W. Todd wrote an interesting paper entitled "The Errors of Medicine." Among his numerous examples he referred to the treatment of barbiturate poisoning, and he criticized the methods then in use. "There are peculiar difficulties in obtaining evidence of the value of remedies for barbiturate poisoning. For among 100 affected patients, 90 or more will probably recover without treatment, and perhaps 4 or 5 have taken so large a dose that no treatment will save them. So in only a very small proportion of patients does treatment matter. If there were a consistently successful remedy for these few, a large controlled series would be necessary to demonstrate it. If a remedy, in fact, only saves some of them, proof of its value is almost impossible to reach."[17]

When "proof" is so difficult to achieve in the 1980s, we must have tolerance for the physicians of the earlier periods. We must also remember at all times that what is true of "most" cases does not necessarily apply to any one particular case. Let no present-day physician denigrate the practice of blood-letting unless, in his own therapeutics, he does not explain his successes and failures as did the phlebotomists.

*HOW DO YOU KNOW?*

## CHAPTER 12

# What Is a Fact?

*Medical students are inundated with facts.* Each course in the curriculum has its own huge text crammed with facts. The faculty emphasizes the sacredness of facts through the so-called true-false or objective examination, where for every question there is a right answer and a wrong answer. The students get sensitized to all this and become uneasy if a lecturer makes a statement running counter to what the text declared or what some other lecturer has said. If facts do not hold still, where will the student find stability? Yet neither students nor faculty show much interest in the basic question, "What *is* a fact?"

## I

In medicine a special craving for facts became prominent in the early part of the 19th century. Among the ancients there had long been disputes between the empiricists, who relied on experience, and the rationalists, who relied on reason. Until the Renaissance the devotees of reason held the upper hand, and in the 18th century theory and reason still played a dominant role. A small amount of fact could—and did—give rise to a large amount of theory, much as, in an amusement center, a small amount of sugar powder gets transformed into a huge but insubstantial mass of "cotton candy." Children love it, but, as soon as they bite into it, the substance seems to melt away.

In the 18th century much of medical theory had this airy insubstantial quality, called hypothesis (in a highly pejorative sense). Yet by the middle of the century a reaction was already setting in. Theorists became less devoted to large-scale explanations and more interested in smaller areas of study. There developed a greater regard for observation. In medicine this concern received special impetus from the Paris physicians of the early 19th century.

In 1826 a French physician, Louis Martinet (1795-1875), published a small volume, translated into English with the title *Manual of Pathology*.[1] This book did not really discuss pathology as we understand it today, but rather comprised "The symptoms, diagnosis, and morbid characters of diseases: together with an exposition of the different methods of examination. . . ." It is really a book of clinical diagnosis with a background of factual observations, chiefly in pathology. Throughout, the author stressed the importance of facts, observations, and the "natural history" of disease. To indicate what was "actually there" as part of nature, Martinet used the words "symptoms," "phenomena," and "circumstances," all as more or less synonymous with facts.

"Medicine, which may be termed a science of facts, is indebted for its present distinction to observation. . . ." Again, "It is not sufficient merely to observe the phenomena which they [the diseases] present during their progress; they must be observed accurately." Again, "The observer . . . should be free from prejudice and prepossession, if he wishes to avoid giving to his observations an erroneous direction. . . . He should see things as they really are, not as he may wish them to be." And as a last quotation: "The facts which observation presents should be collected with care, method, and discrimination."[2]

The import of these brief quotations is clear. Facts were regarded in Baconian fashion as something *there*, objective, inert, waiting to be observed and recorded, comparable to the collecting of shells or pebbles at the seashore. The observer should gather them, classify them, put them away in little boxes neatly labelled. Then he knows where they are—ready for whatever use he might have in mind.

Martinet's text is replete with data—i.e., facts. As an instance I quote from his description of tuberculosis: "Tubercles, in their first stage, present themselves in the form of small semi-transparent granules of a grayish colour, or sometimes almost colourless and transparent, their size being usually about that of a millet seed. . . ."³ This is certainly an admirable statement of what is *there*. What he has written is *fact*.

There are, however, some special features that deserve comment. What Martinet has described refers not to any single tubercle but to tubercles in general, to all tubercles in the same stage of development. He was describing a class, not an individual. In effect he was saying, "This is the way tubercles look, and it does not make any difference whether it is in a man, a woman, or a child, whether in France, or England or in Prussia." He gave a generalized description of early tubercles.

Because Martinet was describing a class, his description applies not only to times past but to the future as well. He has attended to the similarities found in many individuals and not to the peculiarities that might characterize any single case. He is thus predicting the future as well as describing the past.

In America a somewhat more detailed enshrinement of facts was offered by Elisha Bartlett (1804-1855). In 1844 he laid down certain principles in rather compact fashion. "All medical science," he said, "consists in ascertained facts, or phenomena, or events: with their relations to other facts, or phenomena, or events: the whole classified, and arranged." Noteworthy here is the apparent equivalence of facts, phenomena, and events.⁴

This book is a major elaboration of an earlier smaller work, of 1841, from which I take the following quotations on tuberculosis: "Observation seems to have established the fact, that in about two thirds of the cases of tuberculous phthisis, the morbid desposition (sic) *begins* in the left lung. This *predilection*, then, of the morbid element for the left lung, may be considered, properly enough, a *law of pathology*. . . ." And, again: "Another pathological law of this disease is, that the tubercle manifests a strong predilection for the summit of the lungs. . . . Such is the phenomenon, ascertained by simple experience."⁵

Only observation can ascertain the "facts, phenomena, and events, with their relationships" that comprise science. The laws of medical science, Bartlett said, consist of "an absolute and rigorous generalization of some of the facts, phenomena, events, or relationships. . . ." Then he went on, "The actual ascertainable laws, or principles, of medical science are, for the most part, not absolute but approximate."[6]

Bartlett, by emphasizing the concept of "law," is emphasizing generalization and the future reference of his description. He is saying that in any case of tuberculosis the data observed in the past will hold good in the future. This is the essence of "law." In good empirical fashion he stressed further that the law is only approximate. Reliance, however, even though it cannot be absolute, is sufficient to allow a reasonable assurance.

For the medical writers of the early 19th century, facts took the form of generalizations that applied broadly. Physicians were concerned with the way that a disease would manifest itself—not in any single or unique case but in all cases. Such is the essence of science—concern with the generalization and the class, not with the unique individual.

There are some disturbing difficulties in Bartlett's account. Are facts and events synonymous? Are facts and relationships equally a matter of observation? Does "fact" refer to the phenomenon or to the relationship or to the law or to all three? The basic question, "What is a fact?" is one to which neither Martinet nor Bartlett gave a clear answer.

Everyday experience teaches us many facts that guide our actions. We know that the sun will rise, that water flows downhill, that fire burns. Other facts, more recondite, we ordinarily learn from books—that the earth revolves around the sun, that the heart is a pump, that morphine relieves pain, that insulin lowers blood sugar.

Bartlett would have said that these statements stand for repeated observations, generalized. Each statement rests on a succession of individual experiences, summated and expressed as a sort of "law." Scientific facts thus derive from many individual experiences and have both a backward and a forward reference. Implied, of course, is a faith in the uniformity of nature, that what has happened in the past will happen again in the future if the circumstances are similar.

When we study the facts, as Martinet or Bartlett understood

them, we appreciate the element of abstraction. "Fire burns" refers not to a single event but to innumerable experiences of different people under different circumstances. In all instances there was at least the one common feature, and this, abstracted from the total experience of all the people, gives rise to the statement, "Fire burns."

"Fire burns" is a fact. It is also an abstraction, a generalization (with exceptions), a "law," and a connecting link to a whole series of other facts, laws, predictions, all of which interdigitate widely. "Fire burns" is all these things at once. When we say, "That is a fact," we are telling only a small part of the total story.

## Facts as Statistics

Another contribution to the passion for facts came from the growth of statistics. Today this term relates chiefly to the mathematical handling of data, particularly in regard to their collection and interpretation. Originally, however, the mathematical aspect was entirely secondary. Statistics began as the collection of facts relative to political economy and to the concerns of the state. When during the Industrial Revolution the need for social reform intruded itself even on the obtuse, the suggestions for reform were dominated by personal opinion and speculative theory. The attempt to collect data was an effort to bring rigor into social thinking and to create a science of the state. Facts, irrefutable, would provide the necessary foundation. Political leaders realized that the collection of facts was the indispensible preliminary to effective reform.[7]

Originally, statistics, pursued largely through questionnaires and enumerations, was entirely a matter of accumulating facts and of trying to draw some conclusions from them. "Like other sciences, that of Statistics seek to deduce from well-established facts certain general principles which interest and affect mankind . . . it proceeds wholly by the accumulation and comparison of facts, and does not admit of any kind of speculation."[8]

Unlike the data of pathology, wherein observations could be readily generalized to apply to the future, the data of the early statisticians did not have any special future reference, but indi-

cated only *what is*. The information pointed to areas of particular misery, defects in the social fabric. In no sense could the
information constitute a law, but it could permit inferences on
the ways and means of achieving desirable ends.

A passion for facts was part of the general intellectual climate.
Facts were considered objective. They were collectibles that
could be found by simple search. Hypothesis and conjecture had
no place. If enough facts were collected, then for the naive en-
thusiast the differences of opinion would dissolve and truth
would lie clear.

As the empirical trend matured, observers realized the importance of directing interests that would regulate the collection
of facts. Facts had to be oriented around specific questions, and
questions represented bias. In the biological sciences this attitude
expressed itself particularly in experimentation. Experiment depended on the posing of questions, and these demanded conjecture and theory rather than passive observation. Claude Bernard
raised these points in his *Introduction to the Study of Experimental
Medicine*, first published in 1865.[9] The emphasis on experiment
eventually destroyed the notion that facts could be passively collected. But the question, "What *is* a fact?" did not receive the
attention it deserved. Nor was sufficient attention paid to the
different kinds of fact. To this area we must now turn.


## II


*Facts in History*

Let us now consider a quite different area of facts, those which
refer to individual single events—the area we call history. Suppose we want to know who won the world series in 1947 or
whom President Taft appointed as his secretary of state. The
answers to these questions would—if correct—constitute facts.
The events in question are all past. We cannot find further instances, we cannot conduct experiments, nor formulate a generalization, nor construct a law. We are dealing with unique
events. Only when the series was won or the appointment made
did the events literally become *facts*—i.e., something *done*. The

word "fact" comes from *factum*, the past particle of the Latin
*facere*, to do or make.

There is a finality about such events, best expressed, I think,
in Fitzgerald's quatrain:

> The moving finger writes, and having writ,
> Moves on, nor all your piety nor wit
> Shall lure it back to cancel half a line,
> Nor all your tears wash out a word of it.

We have here some ambiguity. *Factum*—the completion or
"done-ness"—applies to the event itself. But we also have the
statement about the event. Which is the fact? Or are both?

An event that is past is like a light that has gone out. Children
are often intrigued by the question, "Where did the light go
when it went out?" The question, however, is worthy of serious
consideration. The light, although gone, may have left some
traces. For example, the closet light may have a pull chain, at
the end of which may be a disc or other object that will fluoresce
after exposure to light. If the light has been on for more than
a few minutes and then turned off, the fluorescent substance will
have absorbed enough energy to glow in the dark. This fluorescence I call a "trace" left by the light.

Then, too, the bulb gave off a considerable quantity of heat.
Delicate instruments might be able to detect the rise in temperature in the room, resulting from the light having been on.
This generation of heat, detected before it was dissipated, would
constitute another trace of the original event.

I am drawing a distinction between an event—the light
turned on for, say, a half-hour—and the traces left by that event
after the light was turned off. We might perhaps say that the
traces are really a *continuation* of the event, so that the separation
into event and trace is artificial. This objection is valid, and as
a matter of metaphysics I agree that we should not interrupt the
continuity between an event and its traces. But as a matter of
practical discourse a separation simplifies the discussion.

Another example of an event and its traces we find in paleon-
tology. We see a fossil, once a living creature but now only a
trace. What we note may be an actual part of the original ani-

mal, preserved by various chemical and physical changes, or it may represent a structure from which all of the original material has gone but with the pattern still preserved, as in a mould. The living original was the event, the fossil is the trace. In the rocks we find only the trace.

If we distinguish thus between the event and the trace, we can ask, "What are we referring to when we speak of a fact?" The event itself—whether the extinguished light or the living animal or plant—is gone beyond recall. We deal only with what that event has left behind—the fluorescence in the one case, the fossil in the other. The latter offers better scope for analysis.

The fossil is an object. Concerning that object we can make a whole series of statements. We can say, "This is a rock; this is a piece of limestone; this is limestone of the Ordovician period; this limestone contains a fossil; this fossil is a trilobite." None of these statements contradicts any of the others, and each of them would be a fact.

For any given object a large number of facts can be predicated. Some are obvious—"This is a rock." Further statements, i.e., additional facts, may require special knowledge. Not everyone can identify limestone, nor recognize a fossil, nor distinguish the kind of fossil, nor calculate the approximate age of the specimen. Although everyone would accept the fact, "This is a rock," the other facts would rest on the word of persons with special knowledge who have studied traces, noted and evaluated the findings, and made statements that we accept. If we do not have expert knowledge of our own, we ordinarily will take the word of someone who we believe has such expert knowledge. These persons serve as authorities, provided we encounter no contrary evidence that casts doubt on their statements.

An object, after it has been studied, may give rise to statements that constitute its meaning. The deciphering of this meaning, i.e., the interpretation of the trace, may require expert knowledge. Something may have no significance to one person but a rich and fruitful meaning to someone else. We need think only of a book in a foreign language, which conveys nothing to anyone who does not know the language.

Let us now apply these concepts to an historical event. There is a fine classical and much-used example: Julius Caesar crossed the Rubicon in 49 B.C. Well, so have a great many other people, before and since. The importance of Caesar's action lies in the special relationships that attended his crossing. The bare statement is, indeed, a fact, but, as Carl Becker said, it "has strings tied to it. . . . It is tied by these strings to innumerable other facts." And unless we appreciate these connections the fact has no significance. The mere statement does not mean anything "except as it is absorbed into the complex web of circumstances which brought it into being." What was this web, this total event, of which the crossing formed a part?

When Caesar crossed the river, he thereby defied the express command of the Roman senate, and initiated the civil war that changed the whole course of Roman history—and, of course, led to his own assassination. The apparently simple statement entails a vast complex of meaning. The more we know about Roman history, the more meaningful is the fact that Caesar crossed the Rubicon. And to one who knows no Roman history at all, the fact has no more significance than the statement, "Caesar was a man." A suitable response might be, "So what?" But even if we do not connect the crossing with the other data of Roman history, the "simple" fact has its own level of complexity. It is, in Becker's words, "a generalization of a thousand and one simpler facts which we do not for the moment care to use."

For example—again to use Becker's words—Caesar did not cross the river by himself but with his army. And this crossing includes "many acts and many words and many thoughts of many men." If James Joyce were describing the event, "it would no doubt require a book of 794 pages to present this one fact that Caesar crossed the Rubicon." And that would be only a partial presentation of the total event in all its complexity.[10]

Here we distinguish the event from the fact. Caesar's crossing of the Rubicon was an event. The statement that he did so is the fact. David Hackett Fischer has expressed this pithily: "An *event* is understood as any past happening. A *fact* is a true descriptive statement about past events."[11] I would, however, in-

troduce an intermediate step. Our statements about past events
do not derive directly from the event itself, which is forever
beyond our direct knowledge. Our statements are mediated
through the traces that the event has left. In history, *what we
call a fact is the interpretation of some trace* that leads us to make
a statement about the original event. Traces must be studied and
be evaluated. Otherwise we cannot make significant statements.

What, then, are the traces of historical events? We have, for
example, various buildings, statues, monuments, coins, utensils,
artefacts of various sorts. Other traces are linguistic; we call
them "documents." Some are personal, such as memories reduced to writing as in letters or diaries or transcribed inter-
views; others are less personal, such as inscriptions, proclama-
tions, charters, records, and the like. These, in the aggregate,
comprise the primary sources by which we learn about historical
events, and by studying these traces the historian makes statements that refer to the original events. Thereby he enunciates
facts.

In history we must distinguish several aspects. First is the
event itself that has disappeared into the past. We cannot know
it in any direct fashion, but we try to reconstruct it from its
traces. These traces, the second aspect, persist into the present,
patient and dumb but capable of revealing much when suitably
interpreted. As a third aspect someone must examine and interpret them, to convert them into something meaningful. *When
the historian has reached an interpretation, his statements comprise
the historical facts.*

Facts, like letters of the alphabet, have no significance unless
they are combined. If we elaborate Becker's metaphor, the historian pursues the strings attached to individual facts, finds out
where they lead, makes contact with other facts (which also have
their strings), and ultimately ties them together to *reconstruct* the
original event. Some events are well documented, which means
that there are abundant traces, while for other events the traces
are scanty. But in either case the actual combination, the reconstruction, has a large subjective component.

Historians study all manner of events, large and small. In all, however, there is the same step-wise procedure—the finding, examining, and evaluating the traces, enunciating the statements called facts, and reconstructing the total event. A biography, for instance, is a good example of the total event.

Biography, archeology, and historical geology all show similarities. There are obvious differences, but the procedure that I call the essential historical method is the same. In all, the goal is reconstruction, through the study of traces, of an event, itself gone beyond recall. The event is not the fact. The facts are the statements derived from study of traces. The best we can do is offer an interpretative reconstruction of the event.

That every generation rewrites history is a truism, within certain limits. Historians do dispute with each other, but not in all respects. Some statements seem beyond dispute. "Historians may come to regard certain well-established historical reports as historical fact, not because these reports are true beyond any doubt, but because there is a sufficient agreement about their truth to dry up controversy. We claim that a report is a fact because enough available evidence supports it for us to believe that future research would neither increase nor decrease our confidence in the report." Gardner phrases the comparable idea, that some historical statements "have attained a status so strongly supported by evidence . . . that to deny them would be equivalent to making nonsense of large portions of history."[12]

The reliability of statements is proportional to the general agreement that they elicit. Ordinarily, *assertions will stand as facts if there is no evidence to the contrary*—if not contradicted by other statements or happenings, and not disputed by those who are competent to hold an opinion on the subject. It follows that a statement may be accepted at one time and later disproved.

III

*Facts in Science*

History deals with events that have gone by and never will recur, but events can be regarded in different ways. Julius Caesar and W. E. Gladstone are obviously unique. Peking man or Java man, however, represent not unique persons but members of distinct classes. Our interest here lies not with the unknown owner of this jawbone or that calvarium but with the class of individuals of which the unknown was a member. So, too, in a sense, with historical geology. The Grand Tetons are an individual mountain range and the events leading to their formation are a part of earth history. But the same forces acted on other mountain ranges. We can regard the geologist as reconstructing a class of events.

I hold this basic principle: history deals with individuals, while science deals with classes. So far as history does deal with classes and generalizations, it partakes of science; so far as science deals with unique instances, it partakes of history. And, in both of them, facts refer to statements about traces.

Let us explore the relation of history and science by reference to an important achievement in medicine. In Chapter 2 we saw how Villemin proved that tuberculosis was a transmissible disease. This is now a universally accepted fact. How did the fact come into being?

Villemin, as an experimentalist, wanted to answer the question, "Is tuberculosis transmissible?" To find an answer he took material from both human patients and sick animals and injected it into other animals. Each separate experiment was an event in history that could never be exactly duplicated. The conjunction of animal, time, place, activity, injection, and subsequent course was unique, just as much as was the event, Caesar crossed the Rubicon.

Each experiment had its manifestations and its traces. Villemin, who performed dozens of experiments, had no interest in reconstructing any of the original events—i.e., the inoculation of the guinea pigs. He attended to certain of the traces, but for a totally different purpose. He was not making a reconstruction of something in the past, but rather was looking forward to the future. He wanted to make a general statement with a future reference, to *construct* a generalization, *not reconstruct* a particular event in the past.

His generalization, "tuberculosis is a transmissible disease," we accept as a fact. Actually, it is an inference, an inductive leap, a construction. It goes forward to something new, something not given in the original data. The facts Villemin had accumulated permitted an *extrapolation* from what he had observed to what he had not observed but only anticipated. The inductive generalization we now accept as "fact." It arouses no dispute, any more than does the statement that Caesar crossed the Rubicon. The comments of Lichtman and French on historical facts apply equally to this scientific fact.

Generalizations that we accept as scientific fact are constructions based on evidence, constructions that indicate what has taken place in the past and what will take place in the future. The generalization, with its future reference, is of a different order from the historical statement that says, "This experimental animal showed at autopsy tubercles in a certain distribution."

In science we have three kinds of statements. First and simplest is the pronouncement about individual traces in particular circumstances—e.g., the presence of tubercles in the experimental animals. Second, through selection and abstraction, there arises the low-level generalization, the inductive leap, or extrapolation, such as, tuberculosis is a transmissible disease. And, third, there is progressive rational elaboration, further abstraction and synthesis, to provide a theory, or explanation of events. The theory renders orderly the individual concrete statements and provides them with an acceptable logical connection. We can regard it as a high-level generalization. We thus have three levels wherein the term fact has meaning: individual events, simple generalizations, and theories. Common to all is the concept that a fact is a statement that arouses no controversy among those qualified to give an opinion.

In science the chief interest lies with explanatory theories. The accumulation of descriptive or narrative facts and the propounding of simple generalizations are only steps toward the main goal of finding a broad explanatory theory. We should now note the relationship of fact, in its broad sense, to theory.

*Fact and Theory*

In popular usage fact often contrasts with theory, but in two quite opposite fashions: the first quite derogatory to theory, the second, highly favorable. The first mode I can illustrate by an actual happening. During a television program one of the interrupting advertisements had to do with a particular health product. First came the presentation of special virtues and claims. Then the scene changed to an elderly, benevolent, scholarly-looking man with a massive head of white hair, not unlike Einstein's. In a slightly foreign accent he offered this punch line in regard to the claims: "And that is not just theory, that is *fact*."

In this context fact was something firm, reliable, and true, while theory stood for something speculative and undependable. If we think of fact as a firm rock, then theory would be shifting quicksand.

In the second usage theory fares much better. As the product of reason, theory is the backbone of science. Through reason man achieves concepts that penetrate into the very essence of the universe and give power almost unlimited. Scientific theory creates atom bombs, makes possible visits to the moon, and brings about innumerable blessings.

According to the first view, theory is the domain of woolly-headed impractical thinkers who lack contact with the real world. The second usage attends to the manipulations and control that theories make possible. The theories have merit insofar as they work, and by their works are they judged. This second view does not address the same problems as the first. The opposition stems from an implicit assumption: that facts and theories are somehow independent. Facts are *there*. They determine the validity of theories. Theories are *here*, in our hands, and quite distinct from the facts. This notion, however plausible, leaves out of account the important point: that what we call a fact may itself be determined by the theory we happen to hold.

We all have seen a magician—illusionist is perhaps the preferred term—who annihilates an object and then restores it to an unblemished state, who creates something out of nothing or transforms one object into another totally different. We see these things happen and yet we deny that they happened. We do not believe what we see. The perceptions we call "illusions." Even when we have no inkling of the way it had been done, we take refuge in the blind trust, "There must be a gimmick some-where."

The very earliest philosophers recognized that our senses often deceive us. If the magician's actions were truly fact, then all the scientific theory of the past several hundred years would be untenable. Our theories impose limits on what we accept as facts. Whatever transgresses those limits did not really happen but is a non-fact. Otherwise the theories painfully built up through the centuries would be wrong.

## Storehouses of Facts

The so-called man in the street has a rather different attitude toward fact than does the historian or the scientist. In popular speech fact is the opposite of opinion. Opinion is something you are not quite certain about, while fact conveys assurance. Facts settle arguments. Facts may be neatly compiled in books, available to anyone who takes the trouble to look. There are encyclopedias and dictionaries and atlases. There are books with titles like *Believe It or Not*, or *Book of Records*, that give the imprimatur of fact to statements that might seem antecedently improbable. There are annual volumes often called Almanacs. I have in hand one that says arrogantly, "Over a million essential facts for every home, school, or office."

Other compendia are also crammed with facts in a different and perhaps more limited context. Let us note a few examples. The Chicago telephone directory, indispensible for Chicago residents, contains approximately a million facts, and every large community has comparable directories. Scientists have their "handbooks," with the millions of facts that we call physical and chemical constants. In the daily newspaper we can note the daily stock-market reports that aggregate into staggering quantities of facts. So too with census reports, economic statistics, the roster of soldiers and sailors, and so on and on and on, list after list, compilation after compilation, without limit. These are all storehouses of facts.

## IV

Medicine contributes an important share—e.g., the data of gross anatomy, those masses of factual information which have been the despair of generations of medical students. The amount of factual information in a textbook of gross anatomy is enormous, and a large part of it students were expected to have stored in their memories, ready at command. This was, somehow, considered necessary for further study of medicine, and memorizing the details of anatomy was a rite of passage from layman to physician.

The student may properly ask, "What is the point of acquiring all this information and carrying it in my head? Why commit to memory what is readily available in textbooks?" The answer is clearly twofold. In the first place, knowledge may be practically useful but only if it is in the student's head at the time that he needs it. More important, perhaps, is the enhanced understanding. Knowledge of physiology and pathology, for example, promote the understanding of concrete disease processes as they are encountered. Other branches of knowledge, as they developed, enjoyed an expanding role in explaining disease. Students will readily agree to the abstract proposition that some factual background is essential for successful practical endeavors and for understanding what is immediate and urgent. But facts are infinite in number; the student's time and ability are finite. Will this or that collection of data be practically useful? Will it make intelligible the disease processes that the physician will be called upon to treat?

At this point we must stress the difference between facts in isolation and facts that have relationship one to another, that have *meaning*. The good teacher is the one who helps the student to see relationships between various facts, who can connect those which are new to the student and those with which he is familiar. When the good teacher has provided meaning for the facts, these then cease to be isolated. Meaning, I submit, consists in the relationships that obtain between a given datum and other data. Facts in isolation are useless. They are useful only as they have meaning.

The financial pages list abundant data on the sale of stocks and commodities. Each of the many hundreds or thousands of items represents a fact, any one of which, in isolation, has a limited interest. But when we regard them not in isolation but in relation to each other and to external events, certain trends may be observed. These movements may correlate with events outside the stock market, with economic and political events in ever-widening circles, and may lead to interrelations that are far less obvious.

The individual quotations, regarded as simple isolated facts, have negligible meaning. The meaning accrues when they are placed in relationship. On the other hand, the individual quotation, as isolated fact, seems assured and reliable. No one disputes it. When the individual quotations are related to economic and political events, the meaning becomes enriched, but the assurance may diminish. Bringing a fact into relationship is sometimes called an interpretation, and interpretations, with their subjective component, offer less assurance than does the simple isolated datum.

Interpretation and meaning are similar if not identical. They both remove a fact from isolation and place it in relationships whose character will depend on interest, bias, critical judgment, perspective, and background of some particular person, and thus shades over toward opinion. There are imperceptible gradations between fact—supposedly objective, hard, and stubborn—and opinion, which is partly subjective and pliable. The listing of the financial transactions represents facts at their barest and simplest, comparable to the listings in a telephone book.

In a newspaper we can contrast the financial page with the news stories. The reporter is in essence a historian, although usually without training in historical methodology. The reporter starts with what he believes are facts. These he evaluates, selecting, rejecting, combining, integrating, to create a pattern. There is a "shaping" activity, dependent on the reporter's interests and abilities. The degree of assurance that attaches to a newspaper story has a different order of reliability from that of the stock-market quotation. But, of course, the news item is not in any sense a "bare" fact, simple and isolated. Rather, it merges fact and interpretation to make a complex fact.

Any given news story is an aggregate of statements and observations (which in turn have been reduced to further statements). The reporter has exercised selection and has shaped the story. The news story, complex as it is, comprises an alleged fact, yet it has a lesser degree of reliability than the simple isolated fact, "General Motors closed yesterday at 44."

One difference between the trained historian and the newspaper reporter lies with the critical attention paid to the validity of statements. *A statement is not synonymous with a fact.* The criterion involves reliability. Will the statement stand up under challenge? Such challenges may come from the statements of other observers or from the unrolling of experience. Most of the statements to which we are exposed never get tested or challenged. We tend to accept uncritically those which have not been challenged and which harmonize with what we already believe. For lack of contrary evidence most statements are accepted as facts, with reasonable likelihood that future events will not bring about some contradiction. The reflective critic can assign to statements a probability value estimating the degree of reliability. In some newspapers, for example, the reports receive little credence from critical readers. Any estimate of probability would be influenced by the reputation of the persons making the statements.

To question the validity of a fact may seem a contradiction. If a statement is *really* a fact, there should be no doubt. According to this view, facts are immutable. What has been done— *factum*—can never be undone. This might give rise to the illusion that facts are unchanging. The difficulty here lies in confusing an event and a statement about that event. What we call facts are not immutable events but only statements. And for any statement we can make a rough estimate of reliability. We may, perhaps, examine the evidence on which the statement was based, although this is usually not feasible in everyday life. For the most part, statements, well attested by knowledgeable authorities, not contradicted by contrary evidence or by our own personal experience, will be deemed to have a high probability, approaching certainty. No reasonable person will doubt that the sun will rise tomorrow, but we will deny that passing under a ladder presages bad luck. And, as an intermediate type, we may have considerable reservation about the statement that eating eggs will promote arteriosclerosis in humans.

The scientist or the historian is trained to test the data for contradictions, search for contrary evidence, eliminate bias, ensure a fair sampling, and use other techniques that we include under the concept of the scientific method. This topic will form the subject of the next chapter. The scientific method has to do with establishing the validity of statements. It has to do with the evaluation of evidence. The scientific method tries to *establish* facts and distinguish mere assertions from statements that are "real" facts.

We may thus distinguish several kinds of statements. There are those which are well attested, for which abundant evidence has been forthcoming, which have proved reliable, and which have been accepted by those whose views we respect and whom we regard as authorities entitled to hold views on the subject. These are the statements we ordinarily call facts. To them we can add other statements that have not been the subject of specific and detailed examination, but have not aroused any doubts in our minds. These we accept as facts through lack of contrary evidence. They are, in a sense, facts by default of opposition. There are other statements that have a low intrinsic probability, that run counter to our own experience and to other well-attested data, and whose coefficient of reliability seems negligible. These we do not accept as facts. Then we have intermediate statements, not so well attested as some, but better attested than others. How much contrary evidence would we expect before we withhold (or withdraw) our acceptance?

Acceptance alone does not constitute a fact. There are, for example, some persons who believe that the earth is flat. There are some persons who are impermeable to evidence. Their views constitute their own private world, which the rest of us do not share. Reality, however, is not subjective. Events do not happen according to our desires or fantasies. There is a reality "out there" that determines events in a truly objective fashion. Reality is indeed objective, but our reports cannot help but be subjective.

There is a crucial difference between having an experience and talking about it. Experience may be vivid, but as soon as we start to communicate it we are making statements that may or may not be facts. We need only think of the variations in the statements of eye-witnesses who disagree among themselves, or the inaccuracies and contradictions that historians find in autobiographies. Words cannot capture events. Statements, made with the best of good intentions, will vary in their accuracy, in the meaning with which we endow them, and the degree to which we can accept them as facts.

———◄═══════►◄►———————

## CHAPTER 13

# The Scientific Method, So-called

*In 1593, in the duchy of Silesia,* a boy of seven lost some of his milk teeth. Clearly, the mere event of itself held no significance, for all children lose their milk teeth. In this particular case, however, in the place of one tooth there grew back—so it was alleged—a new tooth of unique character, namely, one made of gold. This report attracted a great deal of attention. A learned physician in the University of Helmstad wrote, in 1595, that this event was partly natural and partly miraculous. God, he said, had sent the miracle "to comfort the Christians who were then afflicted by the Turks." In the years immediately following, several books on the subject were written, each author noting what had already been said on the subject and then adding his own opinion.

All these fine dissertations, however, neglected one important detail, namely, verification of the statement that the tooth was really gold. As Bernard Le Bovier de Fontenelle reported the incident, "In fine, there wanted nothing to so many famous works, but only the truth of its being a golden tooth. For when a goldsmith had examined it, he found, that it was only a thin plate of gold, fixed to the tooth with a great deal of art. Thus they first went about to compile books, and afterwards they consulted the goldsmith."[1]

Fontenelle, writing in 1687, was a leader in the early Enlightenment. As the name suggests, this implied a movement from darkness into light. The darkness, for many writers, comprised the superstitions of religion, the uncritical acceptance of religious authority, and the reliance on unbridled reasoning; while the Light referred to sound reason based on sound experience. Natural science, which made such great progress during the 17th century, was a feature of the Enlightenment, whose leaders demanded the tests of experience and of rational scrutiny. Experience *and* reason formed a joint watchword.

If we return to Silesia at the end of the 16th century, we note that the report was at first accepted uncritically and then interpreted within a dual framework, partly natural and partly supernatural. In the 16th century the boundary line between nature and supernature, between natural phenomena and special acts of God, was rather blurred. The report of a miracle harmonized with the overall attitudes of the era and was accepted without surprise. Only later did the skeptics want to observe the phenomenon for themselves. The alleged gold tooth, when carefully observed, turned out to be an artefact, not a miraculous growth. The original explanation, although consonant with theology, collapsed before the direct touchstone of empirical observation.

Fontenelle, as a major Enlightenment figure, took great pleasure in attacking the superstitions allied to traditional religious beliefs. He exalted the features that he thought characterized science. Some of the overall relations between the early Enlightenment and medicine I have already discussed at length.[2] Here I will stress only the methodology of science.

I

This little episode in Silesia teaches us a great deal about the scientific method and its development. First we had an allegation, then its acceptance, then its interpretation, then skepticism, then an investigation, then a change of mind with rejection, and then, as attitudes changed, a shift in values. The acceptance of a statement rests initially on acceptance of authority. Skepticism occurs when later experience proves discordant with the statements of authority. Skepticism is the beginning of the critical attitude. We see the nascent skepticism in the child—or adult—who says to an authority figure, "You wouldn't be kidding me, would you?" This expresses a struggle between a natural tendency to believe and the vague stirring of previous experience not entirely harmonious with the statement.

The entire intellectual and social background plays a role in conditioning the acceptance of statements. Persons brought up in a religious environment will accept statements that those with a different background would reject. The thought that a gold tooth miraculously replaced a deciduous tooth did not seem strange to those raised in a 16th-century religious environment.

The allegations about the tooth were made during the lifetime of Francis Bacon, whose writings express the methods of science rather than of religion. Bacon had insisted on a clear separation between the sphere of science and the sphere of religion, between the natural and the supernatural, between the human and the divine. Furthermore, he would exclude from the realm of science all that depended solely on authority—that could not find eventual reflection in the concrete world of experience. Revelation could not serve as authority in science, which depends only on what we can directly experience. This view asserts the primacy of direct sensory experience in establishing truth.

Bacon recognized that the senses were subject to error and by themselves could not penetrate very deeply into the mysteries of nature. The senses needed help and Bacon recommended two aids—first, instruments of precision and then experiment, or putting nature to the question.

Instruments to aid the senses had developed gradually but made special progress in the 17th century. For our purposes the microscope holds special importance. Bacon wrote of this instrument, ". . . if it could be extended to . . . the minutiae of larger bodies, so that the texture of a linen cloth could be seen like network, and thus the latent minutiae and inequalities of . . . urine, blood, wounds, etc., could be distinguished, great advantages might doubtless be derived from the discovery."[3] We must remember, of course, that these words were written long before the work of Leeuwenhoek and Malpighi. Bacon foresaw the usefulness of science, the practical advantages that might derive from understanding the finer workings of nature.

Experiment and instruments of precision extend the range of the senses. Since observation is fallible, we must provide aids to correct its errors. "For the subtlety of experiments is far greater than that of the sense itself, even when assisted by exquisite instruments: such experiments, I mean, as are skillfully and artificially devised for the express purpose of determining the point in question." The senses will perceive the result of the experiment. Bacon had continued, ". . . the office of the sense shall be only to judge of the experiment, and that the experiment itself shall judge of the thing."[4]

The collection of observations, however, is not enough. The data provided by observation and experiment must lead beyond themselves, must be digested, abstracted, and generalized. This task comprises the province of reason, whereas the observation, with or without instruments, was the work of sense. Reason and sense had to work together. Such a combination, Bacon believed, "established forever a true and lawful marriage between the empirical and the rational faculty."[5]

One of Bacon's superb extended similes refers to this conjunction: "The men of experiment are like the ant, they only collect and use; the reasoners resemble spiders, who make cobwebs out of their own substance. But the bee takes a middle course: it gathers its material from the flowers of the garden and of the field, but transforms and digests it by a power of its own."[6]

Bacon did not so much invent as codify the principal features that characterize the scientist: observation, precision, experimentation, reasoning, generalization. He also described three additional features. The first is the need for controls. The positive instance alone is not conclusive, but we must search diligently for the negative instances as well. Again he provided a striking comparison to prove a point. During a storm, sailors will make vows, hoping to persuade God to save them from shipwreck. If they are indeed saved, they will bring votive offerings to churches, in satisfaction of their vows. But the votive offerings that we see in churches do not prove anything about the power of God. Where, asked Bacon, are the votive offerings of those "that were drowned after their vows"? His negative instances correspond to what we call controls.[7]

A second major feature of Bacon's method was the demand for caution in reaching conclusions. We must avoid hasty generalization based on incomplete evidence. He repeatedly condemned conclusions founded on a "few experiments." Furthermore, we must not "fly" from a few particulars to axioms of high generality, but must constantly check our generalizations against new particulars. The proper method goes from particulars to axioms and from these back to particulars again. This is Bacon's way of phrasing what we might call "verification."[8]

In this regard he also cautioned against what we would call hasty reliance on analogy. Inference must not go "beyond the actual experiment. For if it be transferred to other cases which are deemed similar, unless such transfer be made by a just and orderly process, it is a fallacious thing." The inference, the analogical reasoning, must be tested by experience.[9]

Third, Bacon recognized the prevalence of bias and the need for neutralizing it. He described at considerable length those factors which impaired the validity of interpretation. He designated these as "idols" and much of his *New Organon* discusses these well-known concepts—the idols of the tribe, of the cave, of the theatre, and of the market-place.

The chief elements of modern scientific method we find clearly expressed in Bacon's writings. He demanded observation, experimentation, precision, and cautious generalization; he recognized the need for controls, the dangers of hastily drawing conclusions, the importance of recognizing and overcoming bias, the need for verification, the return to particulars once the generalization has been made. Bacon had drawn, if not a precise blueprint, at least careful preliminary sketches for what eventually came to be known as the scientific method.

We may now ask, "What happened to all these fine precepts that today we value so highly?" Although Bacon became the patron saint of The Royal Society, his recommendations were honored more in the breech than in the observance. Yet the methodology grew, became gradually better understood; progress, however, was slow and painful, and marked by many backslidings. I will illustrate a few of the steps, although I am not in any way attempting a history of the scientific method.

## II

In the 17th century Robert Boyle (1627-1691) was eminent in three different activities: he was an outstanding natural philosopher, a chemist, and, especially important for our purposes, an amateur physician who devoted much thought to both the theoretical and practical aspects of medicine.[10] We can properly ask, "How did his overall attitude conform to Bacon's concepts of scientific method?"

Bacon was in no sense a practicing scientist but only a theorist. Boyle, however, was one of the outstanding scientists of his era. I suggest, therefore, that the methods he used, and the acumen he exhibited, represent the highest standards of the era. We must examine what he actually did in the way of critical examination, and not wonder why he did not do something else. To ask why he did not use, say, double blind controls, is quite comparable to asking why he did not measure the atomic weight of oxygen.

Much of Boyle's work related to medicine in one or another form. In his rambling style he made frequent mention of cures and indicated the evidence on which he based his assertions. From time to time he referred to several instances in which a particular remedy had been tried. He referred to the published writings of many of the prominent physicians of the preceding one hundred and fifty years but most of the comments were anecdotal in form, telling what someone had told him.

Boyle had three major sources of evidence—what he read, what someone told him, and what he saw for himself. How did he evaluate it all? We can, I believe, distinguish several types of reaction that tend to run one into the other.

First were the assertions that seemed antecedently improbable, that demanded much more evidence before they could be accepted. Thus, there had been reports of a special stone, resistant to fire, that, when ingested in small quantities, was asserted to be "capable of agglutinating together the parts of broken bones." Although this remedy had had many reports of its efficacy, Boyle remained skeptical and said, "And indeed these need good proof to make a wary man believe so strange a thing."

Or, again, he refused to accept assertions of van Helmont "till sufficient experience hath convinced me of their truth." Boyle did not say, "This is impossible," or "This cannot be." He avoided dogmatic rejection, but, while keeping an open mind, he demanded further proof before he could accept some statements.[11]

The authority behind the statement did not suffice to overcome the doubts engendered by Boyle's background knowledge. Today we might say that the statement rested on questionable authority, which means only that the assertion does not fit into the background knowledge of the critic, who perceives a discordance. The discordance is greater than the weight of authority.

Here we may note the motto of The Royal Society, *Nullius in verbis*—which can only be translated freely. I suggest, "We accept the authority of no one." But this, clearly, is entirely untrue. The intended meaning is, "We reserve the right to reject the authority of anyone whose statements do not harmonize with our other beliefs that rest on empirical evidence." The Royal Society, in rejecting blind acceptance of authority, asserted its right to test all statements against experience.

This, of course, did not mean that the Society actually did test all statements. Boyle shows us the degree to which skepticism was carried in some instances while in others a skeptical eyebrow was never even raised. Boyle gave innumerable examples where he did not question the reliability of the source. He recounted as fact various statements by persons whom he described as "worthy of credence," or "sober," or "judicious," or "reliable," or "experienced." For Boyle such qualities ensured credibility.

In retrospect we realize that Boyle first accepted the authority as valid, and then justified his acceptance by applying suitable adjectives to the source. What a "judicious" person says we tend to accept as fact. But if we ask what made Boyle consider a person judicious in the first place, we would say that the person made statements and provided evidence that accorded with Boyle's own beliefs. Or, we might better say, that made no discordance. The absence of contradiction is a more precise formulation. If the accepted authority had a long-standing reputation for veracity and good judgment, and if his statements had not previously contradicted manifest experience, there would then be justification for believing any new statement.

In his reports Boyle usually trusted his own experience more than that of his informants. When he supported various statements by reference to his own experience, he seemed to make a distinction, based on the degree of his own conviction. For some remedies he felt very sure. For example, regarding the medicinal value of crushed millepedes he not only relied on the reports of others but could speak from his personal experience.[12] In other reports wherein he relied on personal experience we can detect a sense of reservation, of tentative acceptance, with the proviso that more evidence would be desirable.

Boyle had great confidence that many folk remedies, vouched for by the laity, might have real value. He strongly rejected the dogmatism of the schools that on a priori grounds simply ignored whatever did not agree with the doctrines of recognized medical authorities. When impressed by the evidence, he would urge tentative acceptance, hoping that further experience would provide a more definitive answer. Today, on reading Boyle, we are perhaps surprised at the degree of tolerance he exhibited in accepting so many reports of cures. By today's standards he would be called credulous. But when we regard the 17th century on its own terms, we realize that standards for critical evaluation were poorly developed. Boyle was indeed deliberately critical. It is an index of historical change that what to him was being critical seems credulity to us.

Boyle hoped that natural philosophy—for him chiefly chemistry—would prove useful in medicine. The title of a major work, "The Usefulness of Natural Philosophy," indicates his attitude. He fully realized that chemistry, slowly becoming a science, was not yet adequately grounded in theory, and therefore any desire to find a sound "philosophical" basis for therapeutics could not be realized at the time. He knew he necessarily had to remain on a level essentially empirical. However, Boyle had hoped that eventually chemistry, as a well-grounded science, could eliminate the taint of "mere" empiricism. What empirical evidence had suggested as useful might then find theoretical justification. In an important passage he declared:

"For our vulgar chymistry (to which our shops owe their venal spagyrical remedies) is as yet very incomplete, affording us rather a collection of loose and scattered (and many of them but casual) experiments, than an art duly superstructed upon principles and notions, emergent from severe and competent inductions. . . . And therefore, till the principles of chymistry be better known, and more solidly established, we must expect no other, than that very few vulgar chymical remedies should be of the noblest sort; and that in the preparation of many others, considerable errors should be wont to pass unheeded, and faults gross enough, be apt to be mistakenly committed."[13]

The scientist, Boyle realized, must accept error until his science is more precise. To achieve precision there had to be an interplay between observation and theory. Achieving the "proper" interplay was the function of the scientific method, and this method developed slowly. At different times different aspects assumed particular importance. I can touch on only a few of these.

### III

In the 17th century most of the concepts that we associate with the scientific method were already defined, even though in a larval manner. By the 19th century some of the issues had become especially prominent, while the 20th century brought forth major refinements and elaborations. In discussing the scientific method I will touch on four significant problems—the question of authority and its role in scientific thinking; the relation of observation to theory, or of empiricism to rationalism; the question of controls; and the development of precision. To some extent these are thoroughly intermingled. The problem of authority concerns the reliance that we may place in the statements of someone else. In the history of medicine the rebellion against Galen has come to symbolize the rebellion against au-

thority generally. Historians have been all too willing to follow
the strictures of Sarton, that the authority of Galen held up the
progress of medicine for more than a thousand years.[14] According to this view, Vesalius (1514-1564) was the innovator who,
instead of accepting the authority of the past, went directly to
nature to see for himself. Such empirical observation would be
the touchstone by which authority must be tested.

The great work *De Fabrica*, published in 1543, has been
properly regarded as a landmark in modern science and scientific medicine. Vesalius did indeed study anatomy through personal dissection, seeing for himself rather than reading what
someone else had written, going to nature rather than relying
on the authority of the written word.

"See for yourself" is a good motto for a scientist, and Vesalius, as an anatomist, went directly to the dissecting table to study
the structure of the human body for himself. What he saw contradicted in many ways what Galen had described. Vesalius was
saying in effect: "*This* is the structure of the human body. If
you do not believe me, go to nature and see for yourself as I
have done." He might appropriately have used the motto of The
Royal Society, *Nullius in verbis*.

Galen, however, had said precisely the same thing. In his
rather abrasive style he first expressed surprise that his predecessors had made such monumental errors. Then he declared:
"I am now explaining the structures actually to be seen in dissection, and no one before me has done this with any accuracy.
Hence, if anyone wishes to observe the works of Nature, he
should put his trust not in books on anatomy but in his own
eyes and either come to me, or consult one of my associates, or
alone by himself industriously practice exercises in dissection."
Surely, Vesalius might have written these very words in the 16th
century. Could any exhortations be more "scientific"?[15]

We must regard Vesalius not as a rebel against Galen, not as
a knight in shining armor trying to rescue science from the
obscurantists, but as a scientist working in the Galenic tradition.
Galen, although not noted for his tact, was a scientist of a high
order, but, like all scientists, he made mistakes. Vesalius corrected many of the mistakes but himself made still others.

The year 1943 marked the four hundredth anniversary of the publication of *De Fabrica*, an occasion that encouraged much oratory and many special tributes to Vesalius. John F. Fulton, noted physiologist, bibliographer, and medical historian, described some of the observances at Yale: "We had a contest among the students to see who could discover the greatest number of errors in the muscle plates [of Vesalius]. Two students vied for the prize, each having found twenty-one inaccuracies." Then Fulton pointed out: "But these inaccuracies are unimportant beside the fact that this book marked the first significant break with classical authority, and popularized once again the experimental method. Those who doubted Vesalius' findings were prompted to go to the dissecting table to discover the truth for themselves."[16] Fulton failed to indicate that the doubters would be following Galen as well as Vesalius. Vesalius, while he rejected certain medieval practices, did not break with the classical authority. Rather, he corrected Galen by virtue of fresh and direct observations.

Fulton, unfortunately, did not say anything about the supremely important problem, *How did the students determine the errors in Vesalius' illustrations?* Did they go directly to the cadaver or did they compare the pictures in Vesalius with the pictures in a more modern textbook of anatomy? I find it quite impossible to believe that the detection of twenty-one errors, many of them quite minute, stemmed solely from the students' personal observations of the cadaver. When I recall my own anatomical dissections in the first year of medical school, with its required procedure, and the necessary destruction of some parts to reach other parts, it is simply not credible that tyros in anatomy could be able to detect small errors through personal dissection of a single cadaver. Did the students hunt for errors by going over all the muscles *de novo* and comparing Vesalius with the findings in the cadaver or did the harried students locate errors by consulting some other textbook?

Although I have no direct knowledge, the indirect evidence seems overwhelming that the students, when searching for errors, were working not from the cadaver but from other textbooks in anatomy. This, of course, would merely be substituting one authority for another. Medical writers of the early Enlightenment condemned physicians for depending on authority, as if this were something shameful. Actually, dependence on authority is an indispensable tool of science. The important question is not, "Are you relying on authority?" The answer is always and necessarily "Yes." The important questions are, "What authority do you accept, and why this person rather than someone else?"

I do not know what lesson the anatomy students at Yale learned from their exercise in finding errors, but I doubt if it had much to do with scientific method. They learned that Vesalius was wrong in many ways, but did they learn that so is every other scientist? If they learned to check one authority against another, and find out the best way to accomplish this, then they would indeed have acquired some wisdom. But Fulton's narrative does not tell us.

Fulton went on, "The challenge Vesalius throws out to you . . . is to believe nothing anyone tells you . . . until you yourself have proved the correctness of the dictum to your own satisfaction."[17] Obviously, this, if taken literally, is nonsense. We cannot, by our own observations, "prove" the correctness of everything we are told. Virtually all our knowledge, scientific and non-scientific, we accept on the authority of someone else, and failure to do so would speedily lead to chaos. The important term in Fulton's remark is "satisfaction," and this must be reinterpreted, to have a negative import. What we are told rarely gives a positive satisfaction that impels acceptance. However, quite often what we are told arouses a *dis*satisfaction. This means that it gives us a sense of discrepancy. *If we do not note some discrepancy, we are likely to accept statements as authoritative.*

On the other hand, even if we do have some vague sense of discrepancy, it need not especially disturb us. There must actually be a combination of two factors—first, a sense of discrepancy, which is an intellectual reaction; and, second, a disturbance, an emotional reaction, which impels us to resolve the discrepancy. It is all too easy to note a discordance, and then merely shrug one's shoulders. As someone has commented, "He stared the difficulty boldly in the face and then passed on to the next one."

In this respect Alan Gregg has provided an instructive example. He reported "that for some twenty years the pre-medical students at the University of Adelaide had dissected the frog with the use of Huxley's manual. Huxley's manual was written for the dissection of *Rana temporaria*, the English frog. But the students were actually dissecting a frog anatomically different, *Rana australiensis*. In all that time only a scant dozen students had noted the differences between the frog they dissected and the frog in the textbook, and among the elite of those who noted that the frog was not just like the textbook not one student but concluded that his frog was *wrong*."[18]

The students, obviously, had respect for the authority found in the textbook, and any discrepancy they interpreted as a "mistake" on the part of the specimen. The discrepancy, when noted, aroused no interest, no sense of challenge, no feeling that something needed to be explained.

The scientist has an itch to resolve a discrepancy—i.e., to find an explanation. The scientist not only has this drive but also is able to find the evidence that will bring about a resolution. Adequate technical skill must be grafted onto a need to explain a puzzlement. Then, in addition, the explanation must have something we call rigor. It must be convincing. The scientific method revolves around these needs.

## IV

Important in the methodology of science is the relationship between observation and theory, between the empirical and the rational components. In the latter 18th century Thomas Percival (1740-1804), in two related essays, criticized the methods of medicine. The first bears the title, "The Empiric; or arguments against the use of theory and reasoning in physic."[19] In it he showed the absurdities that resulted from rationalism and theory, and thus by indirection praised empiricism. He analyzed in detail the excesses that the rationalists had committed. They "lost themselves in the labyrinths of error," for they were "more

inclined to search after hidden and undiscoverable causes, than
to attend to the obvious phoenomena of nature." Among "the
dangerous consequences of theory and reasoning in medicine"
Percival included the formation of systems. These intellectual
constructs would explain everything through reliance on a few
basic concepts. The systems displayed "an amazing fertility of
the imagination." Quite impartially he attacked Galenic doctrine; the vitalism of Stahl; the mechanical philosophy of Bellini, Borelli, Pitcairn, and Boerhaave; and the imaginative cre-
ations of the chemists. He particularly condemned the procedure
of devising remedies according to the dictates of theory, basing
therapeutics on theory rather than on experience and proved
effectiveness.

Percival's first essay explicitly censured what had long been
recognized as a fault, namely, the excessive and uncritical dependence on reason. However, among the 18th-century syste-
matists each writer regarded himself as properly critical, his
own reasoning as sound and just, while his opponents—the physicians who offered alternative systems—reeked of hypothesis
and therefore were to be condemned.

His second essay Percival entitled "The Dogmatic; or arguments for the use of theory and reasoning in physic." This describes the fallibility of experience, prone to error unless corrected by reason. "The histories of diseases are frequently the
records of falsehood; at least, they contain such a mixture of
error and truth, as requires the exertion of reason . . . to separate the one from the other." Reason was the faculty by which
physicians compared and judged and evaluated. "It requires the
clearest judgment to distinguish them [the diseases] with accuracy, and the nicest skill to treat them with propriety. . . . In
the application of remedies, regard is to be had to the nature,
internal source and period of the distemper, and to the peculiar
habit or idiosyncrasy of the sick person. But this implies the
exercise of reason. . . ." Experience alone is insufficient. The
rational physician "selects and arranges facts, and deduces general conclusions, and thus forms a consistent, rational, and useful theory, on which his practice is built."[20]

If rationalism degenerated into unrestrained imagination,

without the control of experience, it was bad. If experience rejected the critical exercise of reason, and the accumulated generalizations that theory had provided, it was bad. Each modality was subject to excess. For progress the excesses must be kept in check. But how?

Boissier de Sauvages, whom we have already met as the leading nosologist of the 18th century, had a formulation that is remarkably similar to the 20th-century view. Experience and reason have the most intimate relationships and neither can exist without the other, but there must exist a proper reciprocal connection between them. Sauvages said in essence: start with facts, subject them to precise reasoning, draw conclusions, and then verify these by experience. Only in this way can the conclusions attain validity. His precise words: "In brief, only conclusions (*consequentiae*) derived from the facts by precise (*severo*) reasoning, and then confirmed by experience (*experimentis*) can yield certainty in natural philosophy (*physicis*)." *Experimentum* is difficult to translate, for the Latin word may be rendered by either "experience" or "experiment," according to context.[21]

The essential features of science, and the crux of its methods, lay with facts, reasoning, and confirmation through experience. The 18th-century writers phrased these ideas in the familiar categories of experience and reason which at present have an old-fashioned flavor. Instead, the modern temper merges the two concepts into a more comprehensive formulation that we call "scientific method."

The modern view is often telescoped into the popular but thoroughly unsatisfactory phrase, "hypothesis and verification." We can start with data, weave them into a construct that involves inference and hypothesis, and then try to verify the concept we have elaborated. The important but little regarded problem is: How do we know when we have achieved a verification? *What carries conviction?* to whom? and when? What one person accepts as a convincing demonstration may be rejected by another. What seems cogent evidence in one era may seem trivial or irrelevant at another. The factors that govern acceptance are indeed elusive.

To achieve greater clarity I want to emphasize the concept of pattern, as a term that combines perception, inference, and acceptance. Pattern indicates an approximate circumscription within a seamless reality. For practical purposes we consider patterns in isolation, but this is a falsification. Patterns always merge into other patterns. As a simple example we need think only of so-called delayed effects—e.g., x-ray therapy followed many years later by cancer. There is a continuity that in an earlier chapter I called a "trace." Traces are an integral part of a pattern, even though quite peripheral. In ordinary life we ignore most traces (or remote connections), and we regard events and patterns as if they were discrete.

A pattern, then, I consider to be a composite of perception and inference. This composite, for purposes of discourse, is artificially separated from total reality, and then may or may not be accepted as a basis for further thought or activity.

We must firmly reject the concept that any single pattern (or event) has a simple and unequivocal relation to any other. There are always alternatives, depending on what I call the edges or streamers. Patterns, combining perception and inference, have both a core and a periphery. The core may be more or less precise, but the periphery is always vague, extending with diminished clarity to connect with other events. Patterns thus vary in the sharpness of their central core and the intrusiveness of the periphery.

Some of these ideas we may apply to medicine. When a physician notes a configuration of symptoms, he has discerned a pattern. If he notes the same pattern in other patients, he can enlarge the pattern to achieve a generalization. The *Aphorisms* of Hippocrates have long been regarded as a model of this form, which I call "low-level generalizations" and which have found widespread acceptance for twenty-four hundred years.

We can enlarge the patterns still further if we add various relationships that are commonly called causes or causal factors. Historically, different observers enlarged patterns in different ways. The expansion can take place in regard to generality—i.e., application to more instances; or in regard to scope, involving more details. The broader the pattern, the less likely it is to find widespread acceptance. A pattern with a sharp well-circumscribed core and only a faint periphery is more likely to gain acceptance than one with a prominent periphery. Indeed, the more intrusive the periphery, the less general will be the acceptance, for then there is greater scope for alternative connections.

When we expand the scope of a pattern, we run into the problem of negative instances. Can the pattern exclude as easily as it includes?

## V

Until relatively recently, medical knowledge (at least, clinical knowledge in distinction from biology as a science) depended on the individual patient treated by the individual doctor. The patient was sick, the patient received particular medication, and the patient recovered. Does the recovery, with all that it implies, form an important part of the disease concept? This query leads to the problem of controls.

As we have seen, Francis Bacon had stressed the importance of controls. Other early writers also paid attention to this topic. For example, the noted philosopher George Berkeley (1685-1753), who dabbled in medicine, strongly recommended a remedy called tar-water. This he considered to be a specific for most illnesses, especially fevers, but his assertions were not generally accepted. To convince the skeptics he made this suggestion: that the patients should be "put into two hospitals at the same time of the year, and provided with the same necessaries of diet and lodging: and for further care, let the one have a tub of tar-water and an old woman; and the other hospital, what attendance and drugs you please." Unfortunately, this well-controlled experiment, with apparently random selection of patients, was never carried out.[22]

George Cheyne (1671-1743), a prolific author, strongly recommended diet as a major therapeutic mode, far preferable to the massive dosings then prevalent. Cheyne, to press his own method, recommended a carefully controlled experiment: "Let two people be taken as nearly alike as the diversity and individuation of nature will admit, of the same age, stature, complexion, and strength of body, and under the same chronical distemper, and I am willing to take the seeming worse of the two; let all the most promising nostrums, drops, drugs, and medicines . . . be administered to the best of the two . . . and I will manage my patient with only a few naturally indicated . . . evacuations, and . . . alteratives . . . under an appropriated [sic] diet . . . or at worst under a milk and seed diet; and I will venture reputation and life, that my method cures sooner, more perfectly and durably . . . and with less danger of a relapse, than the other . . . under a voluptuous diet." Again, a splendid program, with patients matched for as many variables as possible and with the differences in therapy controlled as well as possible. But the experiment was never carried out.[23]

James Lind, who had been a ship's surgeon with abundant opportunity to study scurvy, provided in 1753 a splendid example of scientific acumen. In this disease many different factors had been implicated as causal or curative. Lind showed that alleged causes, such as salt water, filth, overcrowding, putrid air, might be present without inducing scurvy, and the disease might attack in the absence of these factors. It could occur even if the sailors ate green vegetables. Scurvy affected the common sailors but not the officers. Of the many differences between the two populations he emphasized two: disparity in living quarters and in diet. Modern science would say that during bad weather the sailors lived under severe stress, while the officers did not. We know that stress depletes the body stores of vitamin C. Lind, of course, did not know this. He identified part of a pattern, but could not provide the finer details that have since come to light.

Lind's actual clinical experiments were well controlled. He took twelve sailors who all had scurvy to approximately the same degree and divided them into six groups of two each. He kept them all on a uniform basic diet, but each pair received a different supplement: cider, vitriol, vinegar, sea water, citrus fruit, and a complex pharmaceutical preparation. In a few days there was dramatic improvement in the pair who had received the citrus fruit, little or none in the others. Lind did not, how-ever, jump to conclusions, for he pointed out that citrus fruits are acid and perhaps the curative effect was related to the acid component. This, however, was not cogent, for cider, vinegar, and vitriol were also acid. It was not the acid in the citrus fruit that achieved the effect.

Lind did not find the "cause" of scurvy, but he did demon-strate conclusively a curative agent and a preventive. He fully grasped the need for adequate controls and had the insight to isolate the important factors to be controlled.[24]

In an admirable doctoral dissertation that has not as yet been published, Ulrich Tröhler wrote on the topic, "Quantification in British Medicine and Surgery, 1750-1830, With Special Reference to Its Introduction Into Therapeutics."[25] In this work he studied the gradual development of what has become the statistical method. He pointed out the earlier excessive depend-ence on single cases to supply medical evidence, but he also noted, with excellent documentation, the increasing reliance on groups of cases and the development of the "numerical method," the precursor of modern statistics. A critical spirit was activating much of British medicine and surgery in the late 18th and 19th centuries. It manifested itself partly by the search for specific controls, partly by demands that conclusions rest on multiple examples. John Stuart Mill (1806-1873), with his studies of the inductive method, contributed greatly to the critical spirit.[26]

In clinical medicine the numerical method received perhaps its greatest impetus from Pierre Louis (1787-1872), whose study on blood-letting, first published in 1828, was indeed ep-och-making.[27] In lobar pneumonia Louis did find some evidence of benefit if the procedure was carried out in the first two days of the disease, but otherwise no value could be shown statisti-cally. Louis' methodology was extremely crude by modern standards, but in addition to hastening the decline of blood-let-ting he did much to popularize statistics in the study of disease.

The numerical method emphasized numbers of cases, but mere numbers availed little unless they helped investigators to validate their claims. This could come about through controlling those factors regarded as important. Numerical method, however, did not of itself indicate what was important or distinguish that from the trivial. Choice of controls depended on the insight of the investigator, who sought to sharpen the clinical and disease patterns and to furnish evidence that rendered the asserted patterns convincing.

It is somewhat disconcerting today to appreciate how slowly physicians recognized the factors that needed to be controlled. The difficulty seemed especially acute in studying therapeutic effectiveness. Among the instances connected, for example, with tuberculosis, I will offer as illustration an incident of recommended treatment. Earlier in this century there was a vogue for gold salts in the therapy of tuberculosis, but only in 1924 was a critical test carried out. The investigators chose twenty-four patients, all having the same intensity of disease: twelve received intravenous injections of gold salts and twelve of distilled water. Those receiving the gold did worse than the controls. The methodology seems obvious to us today, but Dowling, narrating the experiment, called it "noteworthy," not only because it eliminated false claims of efficacy, but because it was "an adequately controlled therapeutic trial." Dowling went on: "The lesson was long overdue. If every therapeutic agent advocated for an infectious disease since 1900 could have been studied as rigorously, the medical profession would have fewer remedies, but the patients would have been exposed to less discomfort and danger, the community would have had less expense, and fewer patients would have died."[28]

An ideal experiment would start with groups of patients identical in all respects; then into one group it would introduce a single variable denied to the other. All patients would remain in a uniform environment. Since the two groups would differ only in the introduced factor, any subsequent difference would be entirely referable to that variable. Such an ideal paraphrases the Second Canon of Induction that John Stuart Mill enunciated in 1843.[29] Obviously, this is a limiting condition, never capable of realization. Differences always exist. Some differences we regard as important, others as trivial. Experimenters try to control those factors they consider important, but they may over-look other factors that might be even more important.

Controlled experiment does not tell what is important. It merely permits us to seek cogency for our insights and, in addition, to provide evidence that is deemed convincing and that should promote acceptance. The vaunted experimental method, with controls, is a technique for providing evidence and rendering that evidence persuasive. Additional insights, however, may detect unsuspected flaws. Any fault would lie not in the method itself but in expecting too much from the method. Insight always comes first. The use of controls is a way of validating that insight, not substituting for it. Controlled investigation is a form of technology. Like any technology it is capable of continued refinement.

## VI

In human perception the senses have a relatively high threshold. Any physiological reactions that occur below that threshold will not reach consciousness. Francis Bacon, however, in the 17th century, used the words "sense" and "perception" in a rather different fashion. Sense, to him, meant conscious awareness, while perception referred to the impression that one body or force makes on any other, quite apart from consciousness. Perception was simply the reaction whereby one body takes account of the force exerted by some other body.

With this clarification we can better understand an important passage in Bacon's writings: "It is certain that all bodies whatsoever, though they have no sense, yet they have perception: for when one body is applied to another, there is a kind of election to embrace that which is agreeable, and to exclude or expel that which is ingrate. . . . And sometimes this perception, in some kind of bodies, is far more subtle than the sense; so that the sense is but a dull thing in comparison of it: we see a weatherglass will find the least difference of the weather in heat or cold, when men find it not. . . . It is therefore a subject of a very noble inquiry, to inquire of the more subtile perceptions; for it is another key to open nature, as well as the sense; and some-times better."[30]

"Subtile perceptions" represent the reactions within nature, reactions too delicate to impress themselves directly on human consciousness. They can, however, be detected indirectly through the use of apparatus—i.e., technology—which records changes not otherwise observable. The weather glass—the barometer—that Bacon noted is such a tool. The mercury level (or the pointer readings) can go up or down or remain the same. These data, to become meaningful, require interpretation. Then the readings on the barometric scale become *signs* (see Chapter 3) of atmospheric conditions, and these can lead to wide-ranging in-ferences. That which the sign signifies is indirect knowledge, mediated through interpretation.

Some apparatus might seem to enlarge our knowledge directly without requiring interpretation. Thus, a simple magnifying glass can permit us to see clearly and directly what previously was indistinct. But apparatus can always introduce artefacts. Thus, a reading glass can make the edges appear curved and distorted, when we "know" that they are flat. If we progress from a simple magnifying glass to a compound microscope with its vastly greater power, we can no longer be so confident of what is "really" there. In the early 19th century, for example, microscopists "saw" various structures that turned out to be pure artefact, distortions from imperfect lenses. Progressive technol-ogy recognizes distortions that apparatus can introduce and then makes corrections—usually to find out that even more subtle distortions have to be taken into account.

Technology thus enlarges the range of human perception, but the resulting data require interpretation. The data are the signs; the interpretation is the meaning or the thing signified. The acquisition and use of such data have formed a prominent part of the scientific method, especially in the past four centuries. The interpretations from these indirect data contributed more and more to scientific theory.

By enlarging the scope of perception, apparatus gives us pre-cision to replace guesswork. The physician who wants to know whether the patient has a fever can place his hand on the fore-head and gain a subjective impression. With a clinical thermom-eter, however, he gets a precise objective datum, a quantitative value that eliminates the guesswork.

Technological progress, with its instruments of precision, has made possible the great advances in pure science as well as in the practical applications such as medicine. Nevertheless, the essence of science, I suggest, lies not with the precision or quan-tification that apparatus provides, but rather with discrimina-tion—the appreciation of similarities and differences. "This is different from that" is a basic insight in science. Such discrim-ination, however, requires evidence. Technology is one way of providing evidence that will be convincing. Precision makes discrimination more effective as well as easier; and technology makes precision possible.

In the past thirty or forty years technological advances have been so stupendous that "science" might seem coextensive with modern technology. Such a view, of course, totally disregards history and confuses the basic act of discrimination with the refinements of technology.

I illustrate this with a minor episode in the history of tuber-culosis (cf. Chapter 2). Phthisis, or pulmonary consumption, was an extremely grave disease with a high mortality. Early cases, however, might be confused with a benign disease, ca-tarrh. How to distinguish between them? According to the prev-alent theory, phthisis was a destructive inflammation of the lung tissue, while catarrh was a mild inflammation of the bronchi. The destructive inflammation yielded what was, in the 17th and 18th centuries, called pus, brought up in the sputum; the simple inflammation of the bronchi yielded only mucus. If the sputum contained pus, this would be strong evidence of phthisis; if the sputum contained only mucus, then, other things being equal, the diagnosis would incline towards catarrh.

The discrimination between pus and mucus was made through crude methods offering no precision, namely, putting the spu-tum into water, or throwing it on the fire, or treating it with acid or alkali. The results of these tests required a great deal of subjective interpretation and in any case had a high coefficient of error. Nevertheless, the evidence from even these rough tests might influence the diagnostic decision, which in turn would strongly affect both treatment and prognosis.

In the two centuries since William Cullen was practicing, vast changes took place in medicine, changes in which technology played a leading role. Restricting ourselves to medicine, we may say that technology served in two capacities. It helped to change medical science, considered as a body of knowledge; and within this altered framework it provided techniques for achieving specific discrimination.

Cullen could not distinguish between pus and the caseous necrosis found in tuberculosis. When medical science provided a clear distinction between an accumulation of polymorphonuclear leucocytes and caseation, the older theories became untenable and so did any practice that rested on the old doctrines.

Cullen, however, had an implicit assumption that something was present in phthisis that was not present in the relatively harmless catarrh. And if this material, whatever it was, could be identified, physicians would then have a differential point for making an accurate diagnosis. He wrongly regarded this material as pus. The basic assumption was, however, still valid, and the search for a concrete feature that might distinguish phthisis and catarrh continued. The great progress in science, wherein new technology played an enormous part, finally pointed to the tubercle bacillus, whose presence in the sputum would indicate pulmonary consumption and whose absence, although not conclusive, would weigh against the diagnosis.

We can note two roughly separable aspects of technology. While some types of discrimination can be made without any technical aids, technology can make differentiation easier, or more rapid, or more precise. The stethoscope facilitates the identification of different heart sounds or breath sounds, while a clinical thermometer is a better way of determining the presence of a fever than is touching the forehead. On the other hand, some forms of technology permit modes of discrimination that could not possibly be made without technical apparatus. Thus, the electrocardiograph permits diagnostic subtleties not otherwise imaginable, and so too does microscopic examination of diseased tissues.

How far should the physician carry his discriminations, and how much technology should he use in the process? (In clinical medicine today this latter question becomes, What "tests" should he use?) The obvious answer: as much as the situation requires, or as much as is appropriate. Contexts change. What was appropriate for William Cullen would clearly be inappropriate today. Cullen, when he faced diagnostic difficulties, was working within a given conceptual environment that included only a few technical aids that might help him to reach a solution. The physician today works within a vastly more complicated environment, with huge numbers of disease entities among which to choose and great variety of technical procedures to help him to decide.

The modern physician has incomparably more options than William Cullen could even have imagined, yet ultimately the 18th-century physician and the practitioner today have the same task. After considering the event, each must make a commitment and say, in effect, "I declare that the patient suffers from such-and-such a disease, and I will conduct my treatment accordingly." The scientific method relates to the way that the decision is made within a particular context. The quantity of knowledge and the critical judgment with which that knowledge is utilized comprise two separate variables. A simple example will make this clear.

The grammar-school student who has studied, say, physiology, may take a multiple-choice examination in this subject; so too may the mature physician seeking licensure or a specialty certification. The eighth grader and the graduate physician obviously differ in their level of knowledge, and the questions to be answered reflect these differences. Nevertheless, in both instances the actual coming to a decision, the choosing one answer and rejecting the others, would be analogous to the scientific method. The mode of reaching a solution within a given background would be quite comparable for both the eighth grader and the physician.

Just as science changes over the centuries, so does the level of knowledge as a student progresses from grammar school to graduate school. But at each level the student must make decisions, perform discriminations, and *think*. I remember, many years ago, a child asked a newspaper columnist "Which is the *hardest* grade?" And the answer, very properly, came back, "The grade that you are in." So too with the different levels of science in their historical development. Each level demands its own reflection and judgment. And reflection and judgment are the foundation of scientific method. We must not confuse quantity of knowledge with exercise of judgment.

## VII

Science has to do with evidence, a word that comes from the Latin *videre*, to see, with the added meaning of seeing clearly. The adjectival and the nominal forms show some differences. The adjective "evident" applies to anything that is seen clearly. Clarity exists in degrees and if anything is clear enough it will be "obvious," and speak for itself—*res ipsa loquitur*. For this sense the 17th century had a fashionable idiom, "As clear as the mid-day sun," to describe what we would call self-evident with no need for further argument. The adjective "evident" has, however, a dual reference, to the senses and to the understanding. Implied is the distinction between the corporeal eye and the eye of reason. The latter would deal with conceptual clarity, which, we are all aware, is rarely as convincing as, say, the noonday sun perceived by the corporeal eye.

The noun form, "evidence," indicates an agency—that which makes something evident. Ordinary usage restricts this to the conceptual sphere. Evidence would thus be that which throws light on something conceptual, that permits us to see with the eye of reason. In non-metaphorical terms we could say, with the dictionary, that evidence permits inference, and thus indicates or suggests something beyond itself. Evidence always leads beyond itself, but where it leads will depend on the acuity of the eye of reason.

The notion of inference is indeed crucial. Evidence cannot exist by itself in isolation. An object (or event or "fact," as discussed in Chapter 12) can become evidence only when it takes part in some sort of conceptual elaboration. Evidence comes into being only when someone perceives a connection between an entity (whether object, activity, or idea) and something else. There is a pattern involved. An object or other entity becomes evidence when, through conceptual activity, it fits into a larger whole. What we call evidence then forms part of a more or less coherent pattern and points to that pattern. Evidence is always *of* something, and never exists in isolation.

Evidence is the life-blood of science. The scientific method is that branch of science which helps us to answer the questions: "What will we accept as evidence? How can we evaluate it? Is it convincing?" Mere assertions are not enough. The assertions must be subjected to critical examination. Does the (alleged) evidence fit into a pattern, and, if so, is the fit a good one? There must be an evaluation to permit the judgments of good or bad, or something in between. The scientific method provides the critique for evaluating evidence and promoting its acceptance or rejection.

The original perception that an object or event or activity constitutes evidence results from insight. The scientific method can help to validate or invalidate that insight. In either case what we call the scientific method represents a tool. Tools become more precise as technology develops, but the value of a tool depends on the workman who uses it. With modern technology a first-year medical resident can achieve therapeutic results far beyond the power of Sir William Osler. But is the resident more "scientific"? Osler lived relatively recently. What about a comparison with Jenner or Boerhaave or Sydenham? This problem I will discuss in the next chapter.

---◄ ►---

## CHAPTER 14

# "*Scientific Medicine*"

*Today, if we judge by advertisements* that bombard us on all sides, anything that claims kinship with science has a special virtue that confers superiority. Among the advertisements that preach this gospel I would distinguish three types that actually illustrate three different aspects of science.

One example would be an automobile repair shop that recommends its "scientific auto tune-up." This sounds attractive indeed, but we can only guess at what it means. The sign, I suggest, implies that the shop uses the latest technology, with the latest automated gadgets. These, supposedly, are tools of precision that eliminate guesswork and subjective judgment, and thereby eliminate error. I was particularly impressed by an "inductive engine analyzer" that could perform more than thirty "tests," and, moreover, was "easy to read." Advertisements of this type emphasize *technology* and imply that machines get things done more reliably and more easily than the old-fashioned methods that did not use machines.

Other advertisements reveal a different value of science. We see this particularly in puffs for cosmetics and non-prescription medicines. Some highly touted substances are alleged to contain "scientifically proved ingredients," or perhaps the ingredients have been "scientifically formulated" or "scientifically tested." Here the emphasis rests not on apparatus but on some special merit attached to the *methods* of the scientist. The scientist examines, tests, compares, checks and cross-checks, establishes controls, searches for errors, reaches conclusions cautiously, and these conclusions, once reached, have a special validity. Nothing is left to chance. If an ingredient has been scientifically tested or proved, then it must command respect and confidence. Or, at least, so hope the advertisers. One sense of "scientific" thus refers to technology, with its sophistication and precision; the second sense emphasizes a *methodology* with special reliability.

A third sense, distinct from the other two, has to do with the authority that stems from *knowledge*. The scientist is presumed to have an insight denied to others. This virtue plays a special role in the advertisements that offer, as the clinching endorsement, "Recommended by leading scientists." (For "scientists" we often find "physicians.") These scientists are not identified, but the allegation that even anonymous scientists look with favor on a product seems to impress the public. Such endorsements apparently carry great weight, especially for laxatives and pain relievers.

The scientist knows the causes and the workings of things. He knows theory. He can provide explanations, furnish reasons, allay doubts. This knowledge distinguishes the scientist from the technician, the physician from the nurse. We might reasonably conclude that the public does have respect for knowledge, or perhaps we should say for the person who possesses knowledge. And special knowledge, with its insights into the workings of nature, is indeed a distinguishing mark of the scientist.

These three aspects of science—technology, methodology, and knowledge—are exploited in the all-pervasive commercial advertising, and reflect the cultural values of the community. They are also relevant to the popular notion of "scientific medicine" and the "scientific physician."

We commonly hear of "scientific medicine" and the "scientific physician," but unfortunately the terms are used loosely, with no attempt to specify their meanings. In earlier chapters I have distinguished science, which establishes generalizations, from history, which deals with individual events. A comparable distinction applies to science and medicine. Science tries to understand nature, in general terms. Medicine has as its goal the well-being of the individual patient.

Currently we distinguish "pre-clinical sciences" such as anatomy, pathology, chemistry, genetics, and the like, from "clinical science," which studies disease in the living patient. Clinical science and pre-clinical science differ in subject matter and techniques but not in primary goal or fundamental methodology.

Clinical science and pre-clinical sciences we can readily understand. But we also have something called "scientific medicine." Ostensibly it means utilizing the medical sciences in the practice of medicine, in contrast to superstition, dogma, habit, or tradition. But science is not a simple entity. We recall its three aspects mentioned above—technology, methodology, and knowledge (or theory). Scientific medicine, then, would be the practice of medicine insofar as its practitioners rely on the technology, the methods, and the theories of science, especially the biological sciences.

This seems clear enough, but the confusing feature is the belief, all too widespread, that scientific medicine is something new. Just how new will vary with the individual pundits. Some will say only the last fifteen years; others will go back to the end of World War II; while some will go back to one or another part of the 19th century.

## II

The physical and biological sciences expanded enormously, especially in the 19th century. But at this point we must distinguish clearly between the medical sciences and medical practice. In the actual care of the patient, how much difference did the advances in physiology, in chemistry, in pathology, actually make? At first, very little. Just as in the 17th century the discovery of the circulation of the blood had no immediate practical effect, so too with the scientific advances of the 19th century.

The most direct effect of progress in science was a slow change in the conceptual background and in the understanding of disease processes. This change, so important in retrospect, tended to increase a polarization that has characterized medicine throughout all its history: the distinction between the well trained and the poorly trained.

In the 19th century the new theories required considerable educational background and much study, but how important was all this for the everyday practice of medicine? There was no convincing evidence, in the early part of the century, that the physician trained in science had better results than the older physicians who were not thus trained. No one needed to convince a farmer that a steel plough was more effective than a wooden one. The superiority was obvious. But it was not at all obvious that a knowledge of, say, chemistry, enabled a 19th-century physician to provide better health care.

To emphasize this point we need only regard the divergent modes of practice with their special doctrines and theories, divergences that the regular physicians branded as cults but whose proponents called systems of healing. Homeopathy, osteopathy, hydrotherapy, eclectic medicine, and chiropractic are a few of the better known; there are also food faddists and nature healers, as well as faith healers of varied persuasion. Such groups gained considerable public support, even though their theories conflicted with the teachings of orthodox medicine.

Medical science, however impressive as an intellectual discipline, had not as yet become translated into convincing practical results. There was no good evidence that long and expensive training in the medical sciences was the sole means of making effective doctors.

However, at the end of the 19th century a major change began to affect the public attitude. The great progress in bacteriology probably did more to underscore the importance of science in medicine than did any other single advance. The germ theory of disease captured the public imagination, especially when antisepsis (and later asepsis) made surgery safer, and as vaccines and antitoxins gave hope of more effective medical treatment. The public slowly realized that only well-trained physicians could understand these new developments and translate them into effective treatment.

Early in the 20th century the situation came to a head and the so-called Flexner Report of 1910 marked a watershed.[1] This report, which rested on the merits of the recently founded Johns Hopkins Medical School, provided a criterion to distinguish good medical education from bad, namely, adequate training in science. Abraham Flexner drove home the importance of science in relation to medical education and medical practice.

Flexner divided historical medicine into three eras. The first, that of the Greeks, he quickly dismissed. The second, which he considered the era of the empiric, lasted through the 18th century and even into the 19th. This period he characterized as follows: "The fact is that the empiric lacked a technique with which to distinguish between apparently similar phenomena . . . the art of differentiation through controlled experimentation was as yet in its infancy. . . . Ignorant of causes, the shrewdest empiric thus continued to confound totally unlike conditions on the basis of superficial symptomatic resemblances."

For Flexner the empirics were ignorant of causes, did not use controls, depended on superficial resemblances, discriminated only on the basis of symptoms, did not employ logical proof, and were credulous and child-like. However, this description would not distinguish the 18th-century medicine from that of today. To imply that this described most doctors before, say, the mid-19th century, stems, I believe, from a misreading of history and a misconception of science. Flexner erred in trying to equate good and bad medicine with a temporal framework.

The third era, according to Flexner, was that of science. This, the modern period, he thought was characterized "by a severely critical handling of experience." It also deals with probabilities and surmises. "It knows, as empiricism never knows, where certainties stop and risks begin. . . . Scientific medicine . . . does not cure defects of knowledge by partisan heat; it is free of dogmatism and open-armed to demonstration from whatever quarter."

For Flexner the transformation from empirical to scientific medicine came from two sources. One was the progress in the individual sciences—physics, chemistry, biology, and the like; the other, the development of the methodology of science. This related to the familiar doctrine of "hypothesis and verification," which he insisted was just as applicable to practice as to research. In this regard Flexner emphasized the construction of a working hypothesis and the interaction of theory with fact, which may refute, confirm, or modify the theory. In medical practice the diagnosis is the working hypothesis that may be proved right or wrong.

Flexner went on for several pages, indicating that the much-vaunted scientific method, used in research, is also the proper method for medical practice. "The progress of science and the scientific or intelligent practice of medicine employ, therefore, exactly the same technique." "Investigation and practice are thus one in spirit, method, and object."

The goals were praiseworthy. For Flexner the way to achieve them was to teach science to medical students. Ideally, he thought, the methods—and the faculty—should be modelled on The Johns Hopkins Medical School.

## III

Early in the 20th century Flexner had no difficulty in distinguishing good physicians from bad. The good physicians he characterized as having two features. First was a knowledge of medical science as then understood: the concepts of pathology and bacteriology, chemistry and physiology, and all the other disciplines that impinged on medicine, all comprising the theoretical aspects of medicine. This knowledge, he thought, permitted the physician to understand diseases through their "causes." Second was the methodology of science, "the severely critical handling of experience," just as applicable to the practicing physician as to the researcher. The good practicing physician would thus apply both the knowledge and the methods of science to the practical care of the individual patient. All this epitomized the best in the medicine of that time.

Flexner, however, committed an unfortunate error when he seemed to say that before the 19th century all of medicine was practiced by empirics. This ignores a crucial feature: at all times there has been a distinction between the good physicians and the bad ones. Flexner paid no attention to the outstanding physicians of earlier times and did not bother to reflect on what made them outstanding. I maintain that good doctors throughout history have showed certain basic characteristics that distinguish them from bad doctors. The historian has the task of identifying these constant features.

In any era the good physician always had a knowledge of medical theory and, in addition, he always held as an ideal the critical evaluation of the data. However, the theories were different and so too were the criteria of evaluation. In earlier times, obviously, even the good physicians did not have the knowledge enjoyed later. This lack did not result from willful obscurantism or weakness of intellect. Instead, physicians could work only within the limits of what they knew. Failing a technology for detailed analytic studies, they fell back on "reason," especially analogy. The special conceptual tools for critical evaluation—controls and statistics—developed only gradually over two centuries and more.

The bad physicians did not know the theories of the day, and they were not critical, a failing that the older terminology would have phrased, "They did not reason adequately." The bad physicians practiced what I call "reflex medicine"—a given symptom automatically called forth a given remedy or other response, comparable to the way a tap on the patellar tendon calls forth a knee-jerk. A fever with a strong pulse called for blood-letting, a stomachache called for a cathartic. There was no weighing of alternative possibilities, no reasoning back to causes. Instead, therapy had an automatic quality.

Historically this characterized the empiric. To validate his practice, such a practitioner might offer a simplistic rationale: the fibers were too lax or too dense; the appropriate therapy was obvious: either strengthen the fibers or relax them. To the empiric everything was simple. The good physician, however, appreciated the complexity of nature. A Fernel or a Sennert rejected any simple formulation and depended on the rich and complex Galenic doctrines, while Boerhaave, as an eclectic, recognized a broad range of possible causal factors.

The opposite of reflex medicine is *reflective medicine*, wherein answers emerge only after observation and reflection, consideration of alternatives, discrimination, and deliberate choice. These properties have characterized the good physician throughout medical history and comprise a constant methodology of good medicine.

A present-day medical educator finds fault with current medical teaching, because the students learn "reflexive clinical action" instead of learning to think and to evaluate.[2] I would strongly emphasize that throughout all medical history some physicians thought and evaluated carefully while others acted empirically.

Obviously a difference existed between the best medicine of 1910 or of 1980 and that of 1650 or 1750, but it is entirely false to attribute to the later physician some unique property lacking at an earlier time. The great difference between the good physicians of 1910 and of, say, 1710, lay not so much in method as in the background within which a method was exercised.

This discussion recalls an educational experience I had when a third-year medical student. In a pediatrics class the instructor was telling about a general practitioner who made a house call to a family whose six children, returning from a picnic, had all fallen ill with colic, vomiting, and other symptoms suggesting food poisoning. The overall story seemed simple enough, but the physician, after examining the children, said, "These five have food poisoning, but *this* one has appendicitis." That child went to the hospital and the diagnosis was confirmed at operation. This anecdote I consider the epitome of critical judgment and the application of scientific method to clinical practice.

Although at first glance the children seemed to fit in a single pattern, the physician noted a discrepancy. Scientific medicine is highly sensitive to discrepancy, which then calls for further observation and reflection. These involve two factors. First is discrimination, the appreciation that *this* is not like *that*; and, second, the realization that the dissimilarity is important. After all, there are always abundant differences between any two events. Are those differences relevant to the question at hand? Are they significant? What, if anything, do they mean? In scientific medicine the physician must appreciate discrepancies and be aware of their possible significance.

This attitude was, I believe, well developed in Boerhaave, even though his terminology may seem bizarre. "Reason" was the catch-all term, necessarily vague since it was used in a variety of senses. We can, however, clearly see in retrospect the processes involved. Included were what we call reflection and critical comparison. Through reason, said Boerhaave, "the data of experience are tested, examined in all their characteristics, then scrupulously compared with each other to reveal the agreements and differences." It is reason that permits us to compare "all those ideas arising in experience, so that we perceive distinctly all those notions of which the ideas are composed, and then can judge what these ideas have in common and wherein they differ." And he continued, "nor is anything else required for science than this comparison patiently carried out."[3]

The 18th-century medical writers spoke of rigorous or sound or just reasoning, to distinguish good critical analysis from bad. A splendid example of rigorous critical reasoning we find in Thomas Reid (1739-1802). Reid, almost forgotten today, had a considerable contemporary reputation for his monograph on consumption, *An Essay on the Nature and Cure of Phthisis Pulmonalis* (1782).[4] In this work he was critical of many generally accepted views. I will illustrate with a single example, concerned with the origin of the hectic fever in phthisis. This particular type of fever was a major criterion in the diagnosis of the disease. How did the fever arise? The origin had been widely attributed to "the particles of pus in the lungs being absorbed and carried into the circulation"; or, alternatively, to "an acrimony in the juices, communicated by the absorption of pus from the lungs." Reid critically examined these claims.

At this time there was no knowledge of cells or of bacteria. The designation pus was applied on the basis of naked eye examination, with no knowledge of microscopic composition or cellular origin. Although Reid's critical judgment was circumscribed by the limited knowledge of his day, he denied that the fever in consumption resulted from the absorption of pus or of an acrimony. He saw discrepancies. He did not provide any new data but he offered a critique of the evidence then available.

First he commented on the nature of pus and its intrinsically bland properties. Reid pointed to cases of massive accumulations of pus without either ulceration or hectic fever. "It seems evident that pus in its natural state is not, at least in the cavities of the body, possessed of an acrimonious or corroding quality." Moreover, "to the taste pus gives no sense of acrimony, but is soft, bland, and inoffensive." What the surgeons called "laudable matter, is a bland, smooth, white or yellow viscid fluid; of the consistence of cream, and void of acrimony or putrefaction." In the sputum of consumptives (supposedly composed of pus) there is no "perceivable acrimony." Since Reid could not detect acrimony in pus, he maintained that the absorption of pus in consumptive lungs was not the cause of the hectic fever. If the hectic fever "were caused by pus being absorbed, and carried into the circulation, a fever of the same kind would take place from the absorption of pus in other diseases. The contrary is known to every practitioner."

Reid pointed to other controls (without using that actual word). Where there was an ulceration with pus formation, i.e., a localized inflammation, fever often did occur. Pus, it was thus recognized, could indeed induce fever, but *it was of a quite different type* that had no "affinity" with the hectic fever of consumption.

Reid denied that it was the absorption of pus that caused the hectic fever and asked whether the "pulmonary hectic" was perhaps "a fever sui generis arising from a cause peculiar to itself." His data were not correct, his knowledge was faulty, but his critical acumen was excellent. He realized that neither pus nor an acrid was the "cause" of hectic fever. He rejected claims that he recognized as illogical, but the knowledge available to him did not permit any new doctrine. Critical judgment does not discover new knowledge. It condemns what is faulty and opens the way for the innovators who will make the new discoveries.

## IV

For Flexner, as for us today, "severely critical handling of experience" was an important part of scientific method, applicable to clinical practice as well as to research investigation. In this usage "critical" is a term difficult to define. The word, originally referring to a crisis, has a long history, with gradations of meaning that we do not need to review. In the context of science and scientific method, the sense of decision is important. Implicit are, first, alternative choices; second, the means of discrimination; and, third, an evaluation relative to some standard. The decision depends on recognizing that the circumstances or properties in question do or do not show a congruence with the standard. To be "severely critical" a physician must use the utmost care in examining the alternatives, identifying and evaluating differences, and comparing the alternatives with each other and with the standard until a decision can emerge. The physician who is not critical corresponds to the empiric. He does not consider alternatives, does not discriminate among their features, and does not attend to any detailed congruence with the pattern. He acts reflexly instead of reflectively.

When we speak of acting in a reflex manner, there comes to mind the whole process of automation, whereby technology permits complex discriminations, on the basis of which decisions might be made automatically, to conform to a prearranged program (or pattern). Automation as such—e.g., a thermostat, a governor in an engine, or a Jacquard loom—long antedated the present electronic era, but electronic technology has increased the capabilities to a fabulous extent. Automation, through delicate sensors and complex feedbacks, can, if suitably programmed, make decisions and perform tasks that had long been regarded as typical of human reason and reflective thinking. In medicine, can automation, of whatever type, take the place of that critical judgment which has characterized the good physician?

Restricting myself to medicine, I distinguish two major categories of automation, which I call the analytic and the synthetic. The first provides information but does not directly lead to a decision; the second, through a process of automatic evaluation, does reach a decision.

As an example of the analytic type in medicine I would point to the apparatus that, from a small quantity of blood, provides a whole series of chemical determinations. Conceivably, at some future time a single drop of blood might yield a print-out of several dozen quantitative determinations. But, regardless of how exquisite the refinement, the machine would be merely providing data. The physician would make the synthesis and, through evaluation and interpretation, would translate the data into a diagnosis.

For the second type the machine makes the synthesis and carries out the comparison and evaluation of data. By reaching a decision in line with specific programming, the machine then becomes a diagnostician. A great deal of work has been done to perfect such an apparatus, although at present with only equivocal success.[5] Let us assume, however, that such a machine could become a reality and that we have achieved an "automated diagnosticator." This is at least conceivable. How would it affect our ideas of scientific medicine? Such an apparatus, although nonexistent at the moment, can give us a perspective on the meaning of scientific medicine.

Since the computer is an advanced form of technology, we must first note the distinctions between technician and scientist. There are important differences in function. The scientist has as his goal the expansion of knowledge, usually in the form of generalizations and theory. The technician is concerned with manipulating apparatus in the most effective practical fashion. The scientist uses apparatus to acquire information that can lead to discriminations. The technician operates the machine as an end in itself. The scientist has a sound background of knowledge and theory; the technician has this to only a minimum degree. The scientist must interpret his data, a task that requires critical judgment and a command of scientific method. The technician does not have the responsibility of making interpretations.

The physician and the scientist have different goals. The medical practitioner takes care of the individual patient; *qua* physician he is not concerned with the advancement of knowledge or the propounding of generalizations. When the physician is caring for his patient, he is not acting as a scientist. The practical functions of a physician introduce certain complications in the relationships to a technician.

Let us picture to ourselves the doctor in his office, taking care of the patient, and the technician in the laboratory, awaiting the doctor's orders. The doctor makes specific requests that the technician carries out. The physician, with his theoretical knowledge, knows what to order and how to interpret the results. The technician, who carries out the orders, does not have this knowledge. At this point we can learn a great deal from a broader historical perspective. I would draw a quite exact parallel to the situation in the 16th century, where the learned physician gave his orders to the apothecary, who carried them out in a manner analogous to that of today's laboratory technician. What the apothecary actually did was quite different from what the modern technician does, but I would emphasize the similarities in the analogy.

In the 17th century the apothecaries gradually took over much of the primary patient care, although done at first in an empirical fashion. The apothecaries had learned the practical details that *worked*. They could make the generally accepted responses to the particular situations that they recognized. And they could have reasonably successful results—i.e., the patients usually recovered. In the course of three centuries the status of the apothecary changed and he became a major factor in total medical care. (And today the technician, sometimes called "physician's assistant," is finding opportunities for upward mobility, just as did the apothecary in the 18th century.)

The apothecary, as he began to engage in medical practice, started as an empiric. This, however, is not an all-or-none characterization. The word "empiric" exhibits degrees. For Flexner the term applied to anyone who practiced by attending to superficial resemblances, without real knowledge—a mode that I call acting reflexly. Nevertheless, in medical practice this form of treatment is often quite successful. Any group of practitioners will show gradations in the degree to which they practice as empirics. And, hard as it is to believe, every once in a while a person with no or negligible formal training fobs himself off as a doctor and may be surprisingly successful—until he is found out. (It is only those who are caught that we hear about.) But even many licensed physicians with the proper diplomas practice medicine in a highly empirical fashion.

The physician who wants to practice good medicine will first of all seek relevant data (originally gathered by the unaided senses but now largely dependent on laboratory work). He must also have a background of conceptual knowledge that lets him appreciate the meaning of the data. And he must have critical judgment to evaluate the data. At present, technology provides subtle means for discrimination; theoretical knowledge places data in a framework and defines relationships; judgment makes possible a suitable decision. If any of these three is omitted, we do not have scientific medicine but only a greater or lesser degree of empiric practice.

Let us now assume that the scientists succeed in perfecting the ideal diagnostic computer, which compares and evaluates the data and makes a diagnosis in automated fashion. Assume, further, that the physician blandly accepts the decisions that the computer makes. Is such a physician practicing scientific medicine? My answer would be a resounding "no." Instead, I maintain, he would be a combination of empiric and technician—an empiric because he acts in a reflex fashion; a technician because, as he manipulates apparatus, he is following the dictates of the person with the superior knowledge and critical judgment. Running the machine and carrying out its pronouncements would not bestow any scientific virtue. The carpenter who uses an electric saw is not practicing scientific carpentry. The clerk who punches an adding machine is not a mathematician. And the child who switches on the television set and achieves fine tuning by turning a dial is not an electronic engineer. In regard to automated diagnosis, the practitioner of scientific medicine would be the one who, on the basis of experience and judgment, devised the program.

Practitioners will vary according to the degree to which they exercise critical and analytical powers. In the 17th century the apothecaries began to get emancipated from the direct control of the physicians and to undertake treatment on their own. They may have started as empirics, exerting no independent judgment (whether from lack of knowledge or deficiency in judgment). Many apothecaries remained empirics, but in this respect they might not differ from many other practitioners who held the doctor's degree. We must distinguish the practitioner who discriminates and exerts judgment from the one who does not. Only the former would I regard as practicing scientific medicine. Such a person will have a conceptual background so that the subtleties of different contexts will not escape him. He will examine circumstances, reflect carefully, and reach a reasoned conclusion. When these functions are carried out by a machine, the practitioner who relies on the machine is acting as an empiric.

We must not confuse the use of apparatus with the exercise of judgment. Apparatus can help in evaluation—and this is the essence of judgment—but apparatus and gadgetry cannot serve as a substitute. Without the exercise of judgment, comparable to that which we find in scientists, we do not have the practice of scientific medicine.

V

Through private philanthropy, taxes, and the payment of fees, the public supports modern medicine with its interpenetrating components. It is easy to point with pride to the material basis— hospitals filled with apparatus that awes the layman and often the physician; libraries where journals and texts enshrine past scholarship and present advances; research institutes where new knowledge is being created; medical schools where students are taught "scientific medicine." It is all extremely impressive.

From all this the public has certain expectations, corresponding, roughly, to the imagery reflected in the advertisements mentioned earlier in this chapter. The public expects its doctors to use the latest apparatus and the most recent tests in diagnosis, and the newest drugs and appliances in treatment. The doctor should keep up with the new knowledge, and examine all the evidence sagely and critically, as befits a scientist.

Yet, when I regard the material aspects of modern medicine, with its lip service to science, I think of the passage in the Bible where the prophet Elijah was seeking the Lord: "And behold, the Lord passed by, and a great and strong wind rent the mountains, and brake in pieces the rocks before the Lord: but the Lord was not in the wind: and after the wind an earthquake; but the Lord was not in the earthquake: and after the earthquake a fire; but the Lord was not in the fire: and after the fire a still small voice."[6]

So, too, with scientific medicine. It lies not in formidable apparatus nor the myriads of available tests, nor in overflowing libraries, but in that still small voice that I call critical judgment. This voice asks the important questions: "Do you see a pattern clearly? How good is your evidence? How sound is your reasoning? Can you support your inferences with the means at your disposal? What are the alternatives? What hangs on your decision?" This voice, I believe, goes to the heart of scientific medicine. It has been speaking throughout the ages, but physicians do not always listen. And those who do not listen are empirics, regardless of the technical facilities at their command.

# EPILOGUE

*Just as M. Jourdain was extremely surprised* to learn that he had been speaking prose all his life without knowing it, so too the modern physician might be equally surprised to learn that he constantly deals with philosophy. I do not mean formidable technical subjects like symbolic logic or epistemology but rather the familiar concepts that relate to everyday medical activities. Thus, physicians—and laymen too—speak of the *healthy* child, a *normal* blood count, the *signs* of pneumonia, the *diagnosis* of cancer, the *cause* of malaria, the wonders of medical *science*. These and cognate topics I have discussed in detail in the preceding chapters, wherein I also stressed the continuity of problems that extend from the past to the present.

Now I would discuss briefly certain underlying presuppositions that will make explicit my overall orientation to the world—the perspective from which I view the world. Such a perspective, or philosophy, is not subject to demonstration. It is strictly comparable to the views of a poet who declares, in essence: "This is the way I see things and I hope that I can get you to see them that way too. But if you don't, then I cannot convince you through any exercise of reason." I will not argue the merits of my views. I will state them as articles of the faith that governs my attitudes toward medicine.

## I

I cannot escape the eternal paradox that while all things are related, yet we must act as if they were isolated. Any event to which we attend is the continuation of earlier events, but by attending to it we seem to render it discrete. Yet it really is not. For example, a child, suddenly falling ill, is found to have poliomyelitis. In discourse we break the situation down into numerous categories that permit us to communicate and to act. We talk, for example, of the invasion of the virus, or the inflam-

mation in the nervous system, or the sequellae. Yet we are always dealing with a continuous process. Division into stages is
arbitrary.

Practical considerations, however, insist on certain answers.
At what point do we discharge the child from the hospital? How
long should we continue therapy? Theoretical questions also are
intrusive. Is the child ever "cured"? Are skeletal disorders—the
atrophy of muscles and the consequent disturbed body mechanics—a "part" of the disease or are they a "result" of the disease?
How (and why) do we distinguish "primary" effects and those
changes we glibly call "secondary"? Is the child still suffering
from poliomyelitis when he attends the orthopedic clinic to help
him get over these disturbances? Does he still "have" polio when
in after life the weakness of his leg makes him limp? Or do we
say that he "had" polio, implying that now the disease is past
and only sequellae remain? If we give discrete answers, we fall
back on arbitrary decisions and arbitrarily interrupt the real
continuity of events. In "reality" there is a continuous merging,
but for discourse or for practical activity we break that continuity.

As implied in the earlier chapters, I view the world as a
congeries of events and their traces, which pursue an interlocking course with no sharp distinctions. An event would be a
cluster of phenomena to which we attend, and in that cluster we
ignore all but those very few details which accord with our
interest of the moment. Events merge into other events through
their traces. If among these traces we perceive another coherent
pattern, we feel justified in speaking of another event, especially
after an appreciable time lapse. During this time lapse the continuities may be obscure or unknown, and hence ignored. But
we should always keep in mind the dictum: the absence of evidence is not evidence of absence. Medical progress consists, in
large part, in revealing or uncovering traces that had previously
escaped our notice.

Sometimes we want to call one event the "effect" of a preceding one, thus bringing in the notion of causation. In poliomyelitis we might regard the viral invasion as one event and the

inflammation of the spinal cord as a further event "caused" by
the virus. Actually there is a complete continuity, and an intermingling with innumerable other events that have preceded or
that coexist. "The" cause of an event is a myth that permits us
to ignore details that might be inconvenient to consider.

The concept of "delayed reaction" illustrates the need for humility. A typical example is the newer information regarding
cancer of the thyroid in young adults. In many instances the
victims had, years previously, received x-ray therapy for the
head and neck. We now believe that the cancer represents delayed response to the radiation. The action of the x-rays extended
far beyond the brief period of application and this extension
represents what I call its traces. These interacted with infinitely
complex other traces, of other events and states, and cancer came
to pass. In many instances, of course, those who received radiation suffered no untoward late reactions. Then we say that the
traces of the "radiation event" did not interact with other factors
that would lead to cancer.

How long do traces last? When, if ever, do they get extinguished? To these questions there are no answers. When we can
identify a direct continuity over a time span, we have gained
new knowledge; the problem arises when we cannot identify any
continuity. That residual traces may be potentially active is then
a matter of faith, not of demonstration. Nowadays we have
much more faith in the persistence and activity of traces than we
did a century ago. Studies of pollution and of ecological relationships make us much more receptive to that faith.

## II

I regard existence—reality—as a seamless interpenetration of
events and their traces, wherein the emphasis rests on the notion
of unity, expressed in the adjective "seamless." Separation is
arbitrary, dependent on interest (and bias) that direct our attention and thus play a crucial role in selection. In the earlier chapter on facts, I condemned what I called the matchbox approach,
as if facts were somehow discrete and could be neatly identified,
arranged, labelled, and stored. If the inside of a box is clearly

separable from the outside, then we have a fine yes-or-no situation and the appellation "fact" is very comforting.

In my view this is quite wrong. What we want to call a fact has innumerable dangling threads that interconnect with other threads, comparable to a woven fabric. Just as an event has traces forward and backward, so an alleged fact has dangling threads that relate it to other facts. We can think, perhaps, of an endless tapestry getting slowly unrolled. If, in the process of unrolling we attend to some particular configuration of threads (i.e., a pattern) and follow them for some distance, we can speak of events. If, however, we regard the tapestry as static and attend only to a small limited area, we would be dealing with (alleged) facts. I regard event and fact as closely related. *Event* has a more dynamic reference, *fact* a more static reference, but they interpenetrate.

Any aspect of reality that we try to isolate is incomplete and therefore at least partly false. When we talk about truth and falsity, I take a position of strong relativism. What we call true or false depends on context. When in court we swear to tell the truth, the whole truth, and nothing but the truth, we have uttered an impressive-sounding phrase but one that is really nonsense. We cannot harmonize it with the homely saw, "circumstances alter cases." Anything we call the truth is relative to the circumstances. To achieve "the whole truth" we would need to know the totality of all circumstances, something obviously beyond human powers.

As a consequence we always settle for a great deal less than the "whole" truth, and make a virtue of our limitations. However, the very limitation bothered many philosophers, who tried to finesse the difficulty by recourse to God. To preserve the concept of an absolute truth these thinkers invoked "the mind of God," wherein all events—even the fall of the sparrow— were recorded, together with all the attendant circumstances, past, present, and future. The mind of God contained "the" truth, not relative but absolute, and human finitude did not apply. Unfortunately, some philosophers believed that they alone had some special insight into the mind of God. When differences arose on this point, then the situation quickly reverted to the relativism with which we began.

As a metaphysical construct the mind of God would be a totality that contains and integrates all partial truths into one over-arching Unity. Such a concept takes its place as an Absolute that contains within itself all lesser unities and all partial aspects of reality. I want to avoid getting entangled with the Absolute and its Hegelian overtones. But, while we can steer clear of the formidable Total Totality, we cannot avoid the more limited question, namely, the relations of wholes and parts. This is a matter not of philosophic obscurity but of everyday activity in the practical world.

## III

Whole and part refer merely to the more comprehensive and the less comprehensive. A part—something we have separated from something else more comprehensive—can itself become a whole in another context, just as with genus and species. In a given context we attend either to parts or to wholes. In this connection we can think of the well-recognized phenomena such as the figure-and-ground illusion and object reversibility. In the former, two human profiles face each other across a blank space, but, when we shift attention, the faces no longer exist. Instead we see a vase outlined on a dark background. In the second phenomenon we see the surface of a staircase that can perform a flip-flop, toward us or away from us, as we make an appropriate shift. We can exchange one view for the other, but we cannot observe both simultaneously. Similarly, with the whole-and-part relationship, we can attend to one or the other but not to both at once.

This difficulty has had a pronounced effect on medical practice. With modern specialization one physician may regard the patient only as a gastrointestinal tract, another, as only a circulatory system, but, so the layman often complains, no one considers the entire person. Hence we have that new-old approach called "holistic medicine," with its basic tenet that a patient is more than an aggregate of separate organs and systems and must be studied in a total context.

As an approach to treating the individual patient, holism is fine in its way. However, science achieves its triumphs only by breaking wholes into manageable fragments and then studying these fragments in detail. The medical scientist, for example, does not study cancer "as a whole" but limits his research to one particular aspect at a time. On the other hand, the scientist does not rest content when he learns about only one part but is constantly pressing on to reach some greater generality. We thus have the eternal dialectic of science. It must deal with parts and at the same time is striving to embrace some larger whole.

Science proceeds through analysis in order to reach a broad synthesis. However, there are those—among whom I count myself—who hold that unity and continuity are nevertheless basic and that separations, necessary for analysis, are to some degree a falsification. At this point we encounter the practical attitude: the concrete advantages of analysis are so manifest that any distortion of reality is insignificant and can be safely ignored. On this point it would be futile to argue. We choose our viewpoint according to our interests and the context in which we find ourselves.

IV

Here we encounter an important methodological problem. Why do we accept one viewpoint rather than another? In more specified terms, why does evidence seem convincing to one person but not to another? For example, why does it sometimes happen that the members of a jury cannot reach a verdict? They are all exposed to the same evidence and arguments, but some will "accept" it all, others will not. In science we have comparable examples.

In a previous chapter I discussed Noguchi and his claims regarding the infectious agent in yellow fever (page 221). The evidence he adduced was convincing to him but did not convince his peers. If we seek to explain the why and how of this phenomenon, we get involved in a difficult regress. Acceptance or rejection are conditioned by factors that concern the whole personality, and this in turn depends on all past experience. Acceptance of data, recognition of their cogency, depend not only on the ostensible evidence but also on the personality with which the alleged evidence must interact. The subjective and the objective, so called, are inseparable when we try to answer the question, "How shall we evaluate the evidence?"

Similar considerations apply to the well-known aphorism, "Chance favors the prepared mind." Claude Bernard, for example, noted that certain rabbits were passing clear urine instead of the expected cloudy fluid. This datum might perhaps be considered merely a "chance observation." It impressed only Claude Bernard. Why? Because of his total background, with its unique conceptual furnishings. These we can call the "subjective" component that merged with the "objective" datum of clear-rabbit-urine. The conjunction led eventually to a major contribution to physiology. The term "prepared mind" merely uses a different phraseology for that interaction of subjective and objective which underlies all mental life. Any such interaction is unique for each person. In this instance the subjective context was especially important.

This terminology may seem completely obvious, but the implications for relativism are perhaps not quite so obvious. At stake is the faith that context determines both judgments and the actions to which the judgments might lead. Change the context and we change the judgment or the actions. We must not assume that the "truth" garnered in one context will apply equally well in a different context. That assumption is a besetting sin in medicine.

I am forcibly reminded of this when I recall some teaching experiences in pathology. The faculty, with the assistance of textbooks and other teaching aids, tried to clarify for the students the complexities of pathology. Some instructors were extremely popular because they made difficult problems simple and clear. While I also tried to simplify complex issues, at the same time I tried to impress on the students my personal faith: "If anything seems clear, simple, and straightforward, it is wrong." Nothing is simple and straightforward unless we omit and thereby falsify. I tried to indicate to the students two levels of exposition, the one simple and orderly and the other complex and confused. The former has many practical advantages, not least of which was the power to do well in an examination. But such an examination has only slight connection with the infinite complexity of the real world. We must not confuse a simplistic account with reality. The true-false examination is a highly artificial and restricted context for our knowledge. Enlarge the context—get out into the real world—and clarity, the "manifest" truth, give way to doubts and confusion. Reality is infinitely complex. Any simple formulation is incomplete and, in its ultimate sense, wrong. Nevertheless, practical needs—whether in taking examinations or offering diagnosis or prescribing treatments—make it necessary for us to act on partial truths.

At issue is only an attitude. Do we recognize the enormous gulf between "This is true" and "This is true only under limited circumstances," between the simplistic approach adopted for practical purposes and the simplistic approach masquerading as the truth?

## V

My views of relativism cannot escape the ultimate paradox of science, commonly expressed as a problem in "self-reference." The classical statement is, "All Cretans are liars, said Epimenides, but Epimenides was a Cretan." I prefer the comparable formulation, "All generalizations are false, including this one." Logicians have "solved" the paradox in various ways, including the subtleties of Russell's Theory of Types, and Gödel's Theorem, and other concepts progressively more recondite. But the solutions are analytical and linguistic, and do not equal reality, yet we nevertheless must limp along as best we can. And we must avoid the arrogance of saying, "We *know*. . . ."

Because, of course, we don't. We must, however, act as if we did.

# NOTES

## Chapter 1

1. Lester S. King, *The philosophy of medicine: the early eighteenth century*, Cambridge, Massachusetts, Harvard University Press, 1978, pp. 41-63.

2. Lewis Thomas, *The medusa and the snail*, New York, The Viking Press, 1979, pp. 159-160 (emphasis added).

## Chapter 2

1. Richard Morton, *Phthisiologia: or a treatise of consumptions*, 2nd ed., London, W. and J. Innys, 1720. All references are to this edition. Where necessary I have checked the translation in the original Latin, *Phthisiologia, sive tractatus de phthisi*, in Morton, *Opera medica*, Leiden, Anisson and Posuel, 1718.

2. Morton, pp. 88-90.

3. *Ibid.*, p. 89; pp. 118-119; King, *Philosophy of medicine*, chapter three and *passim*.

4. Morton, p. 73, emphasis added.

5. *Ibid.*, pp. 76, 78.

6. *Ibid.*, pp. 82-83.

7. *Ibid.*, p. 195.

8. William Cullen, *First lines of the practice of physic*, 4 vols., Edinburgh, C. Elliot and London, T. Cadell, 1786 (par. 856), II, 359. (Numerous editions of this text differ in pagination. However, in all the editions that I have seen the numbered paragraphs provide a standard reference. Subsequent references will give only the paragraph number.)

9. *Ibid.*, pars. 878, 884.

10. *Ibid.*, par. 864.

11. *Ibid.*, pars. 868, 875, 876.

12. G. L. Bayle, *Recherches sur la phthisie pulmonaire*, Paris, Gabon, 1810, p. 8.

13. R.-T.-H. Laennec, *Traité de l'auscultation médiate et des maladies des poumons et du coeur*, Paris, Asselin et Cie., 1879, pp. 350-460.

14. Robert Hooke, *Micrographia, or some physiological descriptions of minute bodies made by magnifying glasses*, New York, Dover, 1961 (facsimile of 1665 edition), p. 113.

15. John R. Baker, The cell-theory: a restatement, history, and critique, *Quart. J. Micr. Sci.*, 1948, *89*, 103-125.

16. Th. Schwann, *Microscopical researches into the accordance in the structure and*

*growth of animals and plants*, tr. Henry Smith, London, The Sydenham Society, 1847 (German ed., 1839), pp. 39-40. For blastema, see Lester S. King, *The growth of medical thought*, Chicago, University of Chicago Press, 1963, pp. 192-196.

17. G. Andral, *A treatise on pathological anatomy*, tr. Richard Townsend and William West, 2 vols., Dublin, Hodges and Smith, 1829, p. 378.

18. John Hunter, *A treatise on the blood, inflammation, and gun-shot wounds*, Philadelphia, James Webster, 1817, p. 7.

19. Andral, *Treatise*, pp. 443-444.

20. *Ibid.*, pp. 460-463; 479-480.

21. Cullen, *First lines*, pars. 1746-1747.

22. There are some helpful discussions of the blastema theory in L. J. Rather, *Addison and the white corpuscles*, Berkeley and Los Angeles, University of California Press, 1972; and *The genesis of cancer: a study in the history of ideas*, Baltimore, The Johns Hopkins University Press, 1978. See also King, *Growth of medical thought*, pp. 196-203.

23. John Hughes Bennett, *The pathology and treatment of pulmonary tuberculosis*, Edinburgh, Sutherland and Knox, 1853, p. 24.

24. Henry Ancell, *A treatise on tuberculosis, the constitutional origin of consumption and scrofula*, London, Longman, Brown, Green, and Longmans, 1852, p. 621.

25. *Ibid.*, pp. 622, 624.

26. Of the vast publications of Rudolph Virchow, the following are the most relevant to the problems discussed in this chapter: Zur Entwickelungsgeschichte des Krebs, *Arch f. pathologische Anatomie u. Physiologie*, 1847, *1*, 94-203 (especially 172-177); Ueber die Reform der pathologischen und therapeutischen Anschauungen durch die mikroskopischen Untersuchungen, *ibid.*, 1847, *1*, 207-255; Phymatie, Tuberculose und Granulie, eine historisch-kritische Untersuchung, *ibid.*, 1865, *43*, 11-73; Hypertrophie und Neubildung, in *Handbuch der speciellen Pathologie und Therapie*, ed. R. Virchow, in *Handbuch der speciellen Pathologie und Therapie*, bearbeitet von Dr. Bamberger, Prof. Chiari, et al., ed. Rudolph Virchow, 6 vols. in 11, Erlangen, Ferd. Enke, 1854-1876, I, 326-355; *Cellular pathology*, tr. from the second German edition, by Frank Chance, New York, Dover, 1971 (original publication date, 1860); *Die krankhaften Geschwülste*, 3 vols., Berlin, A. Hirschwald, 1863-1867, Chapter 21, III, 555-749.

27. *Arch. f. path. Anat.*, *1*, 172, 173.

28. *Arch. f. path. Anat.*, *43*, 11-73.

29. *Die krankhaften Geschwülste*, III, 595; see also *Cellular pathology*, lectures 7, 9, 18, 19, 20.

30. J.-A. Villemin, *Études sur la tuberculose*, Paris, J.-B. Baillière et fils, 1868.

31. *Ibid.*, pp. 43-44, 151.

32. H. Lebert, *Traité pratique des maladies scrofuleuses et tuberculeuses*, Paris, J.-B. Baillière, 1849, p. 7.

33. Villemin, *op.cit.*, pp. 170, 175.

34. *Op.cit.*, p. 262.

35. Lionel S. Beale, *Disease germs, their supposed nature*, London, J. Churchill and sons, 1870.

36. Robert Koch, *Die Aetiologie und die Bekämpfung der Tuberkulose* (part of series, *Klassiker der Medizin*, ed. Karl Sudhoff), Barth, 1912.

37. *Ibid.*, p. 224. My translation.

38. Hubert A. Lechavalier and Morris Solotorovsky, *Three centuries of microbiology*, New York, McGraw-Hill, 1965, pp. 110-114. The authors, in discussing Koch, provide long excerpts, in translation, from several of his most important contributions.

## Chapter 3

1. Lester S. King, Signs and symptoms, *J. Am. Med. Assn.*, 1968, *206*, 1063-1065.

2. *Stedman's medical dictionary*, 23rd ed., Baltimore, Williams and Wilkins, 1976, *symptom, sign*.

3. A. McGehee Harvey, James Bordley III, and Jeremiah A. Barondess, *Differential diagnosis: the interpretation of clinical evidence*, 3rd ed., Philadelphia, W. B. Saunders Co., 1979, p. 7; John A. Prior and Jack S. Silberstein, *Physical examination: the history and examination of the patient*, St. Louis, C. V. Mosby, 1977, p. 5.

4. John D. Comrie, *Black's medical dictionary*, 19th ed., London, Adam and Charles Black, 1948, *symptom*.

5. John Fernel, *Pathologiae libri vii*, Book II, Chapter 1 (Quid symptoma . . .). There are a great many editions of Fernel's works, and notation by the brief chapter headings is the most satisfactory mode of reference. The edition I used was *Universa medicina*, Leiden, Francis Hack, 1645, p. 388.

6. Daniel Sennert, De Symptomatibus, *Institutiones medicinae*, Book II, Part III, Sect. I, Chapter 1, in *Opera omnia*, 3 vols., Leiden, Huguetan, 1650, I, 372.

7. Fernel, *op.cit.*, Chapter 7, De signis, I, 397.

8. Sennert, De methodi . . . et quid signum, *Institutiones medicinae*, Book III, Part I, Sect. I, Chapter 1, *Opera omnia*, I, 447; Antoine Deidier, *Institutiones medicinae theoricae, physiologiam et pathologiam complectentes*, Montpellier, Pech, 1711, sig. a2.

9. Herman Boerhaave, *Praelectiones academicae*, 5 vols., Turin, Typographia Regia (par. 875), I, 182, my translation. The standard English translation, *Academical lectures on the theory of physic*, 6 vols, London, Rivington et al., 1751, 1757, is in general moderately reliable but for this passage (VI, 117) is utterly unsatisfactory.

10. A. J. Landré-Beauvais, *Séméiotique, ou traité des signes des maladies*, 2nd ed., Paris, J. A. Brosson, 1813, p. 3.

11. Lester S. King, *The philosophy of medicine: the early eighteenth century*, Cambridge, Massachusetts, Harvard University Press, 1978, p. 251.

12. Lester S. King, *The growth of medical thought*, Chicago, University of Chicago Press, 1963, p. 21.

13. Lester S. King, Auscultation in England, 1821-1837, *Bull. Hist. Med.*, 1959, *33*, 446-453.

14. Jacob M. Da Costa, *Medical diagnosis, with special references to practical medicine*, Philadelphia, J. B. Lippincott and Co., 1864, pp. 14-15 (emphasis added).

15. W. A. Newman Dorland, *The American illustrated medical dictionary*, Philadelphia, W. B. Saunders, 1900, *symptom*.

## Chapter 4

1. A. McGehee Harvey, James Bordley III, and Jeremiah A. Barondess, *Differential diagnosis: the interpretation of clinical evidence*, 3rd ed., Philadelphia, W. B. Saunders Co., 1979, p. 3.

2. Among the works dealing with this subject I would mention Ralph L. Engle and B. J. Davis, Medical diagnosis: present, past, and future, *Arch. Int. Med.*, 1963, *112*, 512-543; Alvan R. Feinstein, *Clinical judgment*, Baltimore, Williams and Wilkins Co., 1967; Edmond A. Murphy, *The logic of medicine*, Baltimore, The Johns Hopkins University Press, 1976; Henrick R. Wulff, *Rational diagnosis and treatment*, Oxford, Blackwell, 1976.

3. Johann Georg Zimmermann, *A treatise on experience in physic*, 2 vols., London, G. Wilkie, 1782, I, 167.

4. W. S. Jevons, *The principles of science: a treatise in logic and scientific method*, London, Macmillan and Co., 1892, p. 711.

5. Roger Tory Peterson and Margaret McKenney, *A field guide to wildflowers*, Boston, Houghton Mifflin Co., 1968.

Francis Bacon, *The new organon: or true directions concerning the interpretation of nature*, Book I, Aphorism 122, in *The new organon and related writings*, ed. Fulton H. Anderson, New York, The Liberal Arts Press, 1960, p. 112.

7. Herman Boerhaave, *Academical lectures on the theory of physic*, 6 vols., London, Rivington et al., 1751-1757 (par. 907, note), VI, 149 (capitalization modernized).

8. Herman Boerhaave, *Praelectiones academicae*, ed. Albert Haller, 5 vols., Turin, Typographia Regia, 1742-1745 (pars. 871, note, and 877), V, 183, 182, my translation. The standard English translation, the *Academical lectures*, VI, 113, 118, is not satisfactory here.

9. Gerard L. B. van Swieten, *Commentaries upon Boerhaave's aphorisms*, 18 vols., Edinburgh, Elliot, 1776, IV, 232, 237, 257.

10. (Jean Astruc), *Traité des tumeurs et des ulceres*, 2 vols., Paris, Cavelier, 1759, II, 1-70.

11. Francis Delafield and T. Mitchell Prudden, *A handbook of pathological anatomy and histology*, 3rd ed., New York, William Wood and Co., 1889, pp. 467-470.

## Chapter 5

1. *The works of Thomas Sydenham*, tr. from the Latin edition of Dr. Greenhill by G. Latham, 2 vols., London, The Sydenham Society, 1848-1850 (Preface to the third ed., par. 7), I, 13.

2. Agnes Arber, *Herbals, their origin and evolution*, Cambridge, The University Press, 1938, p. 168.

3. Sydenham, *loc.cit.*

4. *Ibid., op.cit.* (par. 12), p. 15.

5. William T. Stearn, Linnaean classification, nomenclature, and method, Appendix to Wilfred Blunt, *The compleat naturalist: a life of Linnaeus*, New York, The Viking Press, 1971, p. 243.

6. London, Theo. Coates, 1640, Table of contents.

7. *Op.cit.*, portion of title page.

8. Arber, p. 264.

9. Good representative studies are Blunt, *The compleat naturalist*; James L. Larson, *Reason and experience: the representation of natural order in the work of Carl von Linné*, Berkeley, University of California Press, 1971.

10. Lester S. King, *The medical world of the eighteenth century*, Chicago, University of Chicago Press, 1958, pp. 198-205.

11. John Drummond, An essay on the improvement of medicine, *Medical essays and observations*, revised and published by a society in Edinburgh, Edinburgh, 1733, *I*, 258-272.

12. King, *Medical world*, pp. 193-226; Boissier de Sauvages and 18th century nosology, *Bull. Hist. Med.*, 1966, *40*, 43-51.

13. Lester S. King, *The philosophy of medicine: the early eighteenth century*, Cambridge, Massachusetts, Harvard University Press, 1978, pp. 244-250.

14. Francisco Boissier de Sauvages, *Nosologia methodica sistens morborum classes*, 2 vols., Amsterdam, de Tournes, 1768 (Prolegomena, pars. 63-77), I, 18-21; *Nosologie methodique*, 3 vols., Paris, Herissant, 1770-1771, I, 24-28.

15. Sauvages, (Prolegomena, par. 351); *Nosologia*, I, 81-83; *Nosologie*, I, 108.

16. See, for example, Paul B. Beeson and Walsh McDermott, *Textbook of medicine*, 14th ed., Philadelphia, W. B. Saunders, 1975, p. 1402.

17. *Manual of the international statistical classification of diseases, injuries, and causes of death*, Geneva, World Health Organization, 1977 (Introduction), p. vii.

## Chapter 6

1. Lester S. King, *The philosophy of medicine: the early eighteenth century*, Cambridge, Massachusetts, Harvard University Press, 1978, *passim*.

2. Daniel Sennert, *Institutiones medicinae*, Book I, Chapter 3 (De sanitate); Book II, Chapter 1 (De morbi natura), in *Opera omnia*, 3 vols., Leiden, Huguetan, 1650, I, 262, 310 (my translation).

3. Sennert, De morbi natura, *Opera omnia*, I, 310, 313.

4. Freidrich Hoffmann, *Philosophiae corporis humani vivi et sani*, Book II, Chapter 1 (De sanitatis natura, par. 1); *Prolegomena de verae pathologiae natura*,

Chapter 2 (De morborum et symptomatum natura, par. 3), in *Medicinae rationalis systematicae*, 8 vols. in 4, first and second editions mixed, Halle, Renger, 1729-1739, I, 318; II, 56.

5. Herman Boerhaave, *Academical lectures on the theory of physic*, 6 vols., London, Rivington et al., 1751-1757 (pars. 1 and 2), I, 2-3.

6. *Ibid.*, (par. 889 and note), VI, 133-134.

7. King, *The philosophy of medicine*, pp. 182-208.

8. F. Osterlin, *Medical logic*, tr. and ed., G. Whitley, London, The Sydenham Society, 1855, p. 5.

9. Thomas Clifford Allbutt, Introduction, *A system of medicine by many writers*, ed., T. C. Allbutt, 8 vols., London, Macmillan, 1896-1898, I, xxxii, emphasis added.

10. *Phil.Sci.*, 1954, *21*, 193-203.

11. The concept of disease (editorial), *Brit.Med. J.*, 1979, *2*, 751-752; E.J.M. Campbell, J. G. Scadding, and R. S. Roberts, The concept of disease, *Ibid.*, pp. 757-762; Christopher Boorse, On the distinction between disease and illness, *Phil. and Public Affairs*, 1975, *5*, 49-68; *Ibid.*, Health as a theoretical concept, *Phil.Sci.*, 1977, *44*, 542-573; George Engel, A unified concept of health and disease, *Perspec. Biol. and Med.*, 1960, *3*, 459-485; H. Tristram Engelhardt, Jr., The concepts of health and disease, in *Evaluation and explanation in the biomedical sciences*, ed. H. Tristram Engelhardt, Jr. and Stuart F. Spicker, Dordrecht, Holland and Boston, Massachusetts, D. Reidel, 1975, pp. 126-141; *Ibid.*, Explanatory models in medicine: facts, theories and values, *Texas Rep. Biol. and Med.*, 1974, *32*, 225-239; Robert P. Hudson, The concept of disease, *Ann.Int.Med.*, 1966, *65*, 595-601; F. Kraüpl Taylor, *The concepts of illness, disease and morbus*, Cambridge, The University Press, 1979. For information on the Chinese custom of binding the feet of female children, see Ilza Veith, The history of medicine dolls and footbinding in China, *Clio Medica*, 1980, *14*, 255-267. See also the newly published *Concepts of health and disease*, ed. Arthur L. Caplan, H. Tristram Engelhardt, Jr., and James J. McCartney, Reading, Mass., Addison-Wesley, 1981.

## Chapter 7

1. Hippocrates, *Aphorisms*, Section 4, numbers 75, 77, 79, in *The medical works of Hippocrates*, tr. John Chadwick and W. N. Mann, Oxford, Blackwell, 1950, p. 163.

2. Otto E. Gutentag, On the clinical entity, *Ann. Int. Med.*, 1949, *31*, 484-496.

3. Philippe Pinel, *Nosographie philosophique, ou la méthode de l'analyse appliqué à la médecine*, 5th ed., 3 vols., Paris, Brosson, 1813 (par. 464), I, 382.

4. Lester S. King, *The philosophy of medicine: the early eighteenth century*, Cambridge, Massachusetts, Harvard University Press, 1978, pp. 182-208.

5. P.-H. Nysten, *Dictionnaire de médecine, de chirurgie, de pharmacie*, 10th ed., ed. E. Littré and Ch. Robin, Paris, Baillière, 1855, entry *syndrome*.

## Chapter 8

1. Hippocrates, *Epidemics*, Bk. 1, par. 26, in *The medical works of Hippocrates*, tr. John Chadwick and W. N. Mann, Oxford, Blackwell, 1950, p. 43.

2. P. Ch. Louis, *Researches on the effects of bloodletting in some inflammatory diseases*, tr. C. G. Putnam, Boston, Hilliard, Gray and Co., 1836.

3. Lester S. King and Marjorie C. Meehan, A history of the autopsy: a review, *Am. J. Path.*, 1973, 73:514-544.

4. See p. 101.

5. Giovanni-Battisti Morgagni, *The seats and causes of diseases, investigated by anatomy*, tr. Benjamin Alexander, 3 vols., London, Millar, 1769.

6. Lester S. King, *The philosophy of medicine: the early 18th century*, Cambridge, Massachusetts, Harvard University Press, 1978, Chapter 3, pp. 41-63, esp. 43-46.

7. For details the reader may consult any textbook of traditional logic. I have found especially satisfactory the older text, H.W.B. Joseph, *An introduction to logic*, 2nd ed., Oxford, The Clarendon Press, 1916 (1950 printing).

8. L. J. Rather, Towards a philosophical study of the idea of disease, in *The historical development of physiological thought*, ed. Chandler McC. Brooks and Paul F. Cranefield, New York, Hafner, 1959, pp. 351-373; *Disease, life and man: selected essays by Rudolph Virchow*, tr. with introduction by Lelland J. Rather, Stanford, California, Stanford University Press, 1958, (Introduction) pp. 10-24, (Standpoints in scientific medicine) pp. 26-39, (Scientific method and therapeutic standpoints) pp. 40-66, (One hundred years of general pathology) pp. 170-215; Owsei Temkin, The scientific approach to disease: specific entity and individual sickness, in Temkin, *The double face of Janus*, Baltimore, The Johns Hopkins University Press, 1977, pp. 441-455; Walter Pagel, Van Helmont's conception of disease—to be or not to be? The influence of Paracelsus, *Bull. Hist. Med.*, 1972, 46, 419-453; Peter H. Niebyl, Sennert, van Helmont, and medical ontology, *Bull. Hist. Med.*, 1971, 45, 115-137.

9. As I have discussed in Chapter 3, the term "symptom" includes what is often designated as "sign." Symptom indicates any manifestation of disease.

10. King, *Road to medical enlightenment; Philosophy of medicine.*

11. Virchow, *Disease, life, and man*, p. 192.

12. For this aspect of Boyle's work, see King, *Road to medical enlightenment*, pp. 64-66; *Philosophy of medicine*, p. 84.

13. Plato, *Statesman*, 285b (I have used the Jowett translation); see also, Lester S. King, Plato's concepts of medicine, *J. Hist. Med.*, 1954, 9, 38-48.

14. See *infra*, Chapter 12, What is a fact?

## Chapter 9

1. H.L.A. Hart and A. M. Honoré, *Causation in the law*, Oxford, The Clarendon Press, 1959.

2. Daniel Sennert, *Hypomnema II*, Chapter 1 (Quid sint occultae qualitates?), *Opera omnia*, 3 vols., Leiden, Huguetan, 1650, I, 147.

3. Lester S. King, *The Medical world of the eighteenth century*, Chicago, University of Chicago Press, 1958, pp. 65-70.

4. Herman Boerhaave, *Aphorismi de cognoscendis et curandis morbis*, 6th ed., Louvain, van Overbeke, 1752 (Aphorisms 33, 63), pp. 7, 14. The best translation, together with extensive commentaries, is found in Baron van Swieten, *Commentaries upon Boerhaave's aphorisms*, 18 vols., Edinburgh, Elliot, 1776. The quotations in the text are found in I, 77, 148.

5. Hippocrates, *Aphorisms*, Section 4, number 24 and section 5, number 37, in *The medical works of Hippocrates*, tr. John Chadwick and W. N. Mann, Oxford, Blackwell, 1950, pp. 160, 161.

6. R. Harré, *The philosophies of science*, Oxford University Press, 1972, p. 183.

7. King, *Medical world*, pp. 83-86.

8. For the whole concept of the non-naturals, see L. J. Rather, The "six things non-natural," *Clio Medica*, 1968, *3*, 333-347; Saul Jarcho, Galen's six non-naturals, *Bull. Hist. Med.*, 1970, *44*, 372-377; Peter H. Niebyl, The non-naturals, *ibid.*, 1971, *45*, 486-492.

9. Lester S. King, *The philosophy of medicine: the early eighteenth century*, Cambridge, Massachusetts, Harvard University Press, 1978, pp. 208-232.

## Chapter 10

1. Lazar Riverius, *Institutiones medicae*, Bk. II, Sec. 3, Chapter 1, (De causae morbificae natura), in *Opera medica universa*, Geneva, de Tournes, 1728, p. 39, my translation.

2. John Stuart Mill, *A system of logic, ratiocinative and inductive*, 2 vols., second ed., London, John W. Parker, 1846, I, 404.

3. Herman Boerhaave, *Academical lectures on the theory of physic*, 6 vols., London, Rivington et al., 1751-1757 (par. 740 and note), V, 379; Lester S. King, *The philosophy of medicine: the early eighteenth century*, Cambridge, Massachusetts, Harvard University Press, 1978, pp. 222-230.

4. William Cullen, *First lines of the practice of physic*, 4 vols., Edinburgh, Elliot, 1776 (par. 878), II, 384-385.

5. King, *Philosophy of medicine*, pp. 182-208.

6. My discussion of this problem is, I believe, in agreement with Mandelbaum's views on causality: Maurice Mandelbaum, *The anatomy of historical knowledge*, Baltimore, The Johns Hopkins University Press, 1977, pp. 47-108, especially pp. 81-87.

7. Detailed references to primary sources will be found in Lester S. King, Dr. Koch's postulates, *J. Hist. Med.*, 1952, 7, 350-361.

8. Mandelbaum, *Anatomy of historal knowledge*, p. 93.

9. *Ibid.*, p. 67.

## Chapter 11

1. Henry Clutterbuck, *Lectures on blood-letting*, Philadelphia, Haswell, Barrington, and Haswell, 1829, pp. 11-12.

2. Lester S. King, *Medical world of the eighteenth century*, Chicago, University of Chicago Press, 1958, pp. 83-89.

3. Baron van Swieten, *Commentaries upon Boerhaave's aphorisms concerning the knowledge and cure of disease*, 18 vols., Edinburgh, Elliot, 1776 (pars. 396, 398), III, 335, 360.

4. Lester S. King, *Growth of medical thought*, Chicago, University of Chicago Press, 1963, pp. 182-185.

5. King, *Medical world*, pp. 125-127; van Swieten, *Commentaries* (par. 610), V. 284-285.

6. William Cullen, *First lines of the practice of physic*, 4 vols., Edinburgh, Elliot, 1786 (pars. 241, 240), I, 271-276.

7. *Ibid.* (par. 262), I, 298.

8. *Ibid.* (pars. 264, 41, 126, 127, 137), I, 264, 93, 182-183, 193.

9. *Ibid.* (pars. 125-200), I, 180-236.

10. King, *Medical world*, pp. 143-150; Guenter B. Risse, The Brownian system of medicine: its theoretical and practical implications, *Clio Medica*, 1970, *5*, 45-51; *ibid.*, The quest for certainty in medicine: John Brown's system of medicine in France, *Bull. Hist. Med.*, 1971, *45*, 1-12.

11. King, *Medical world*, pp. 147-151.

12. All the quotations are taken from Clutterbuck, *Lectures on blood-letting*, Lecture 4, pp. 27-37.

13. James Wardrop, *On the curative effects of the abstraction of blood*, Philadelphia, A. Waldie, 1837. My exposition derives from discourses II, III, and IV, pp. 15-41.

14. References to the primary sources will be found in Lester S. King, The blood-letting controversy: a study in the scientific method, *Bull. Hist. Med.*, 1961, *35*, 1-13.

15. Guenter B. Risse, The renaissance of bloodletting: a chapter in modern therapeutics, *J. Hist. Med.*, 1979, *34*, 1-22. A relevant study is A. Clair Siddal, Bloodletting in American obstetric practice, 1800-1945, *Bull. Hist. Med.*, 1980, *54*, 101-110. Leon S. Bryan, Jr., Blood-letting in American medicine, 1830-1892, *Bull. Hist. Med.*, 1964, *38*, 516-529. See also John S. Haller, Jr., *American Medicine in Transition, 1840-1910*, Urbana, Illinois, University of Illinois Press, 1981, p. 36-66

16. *The works of Thomas Sydenham*, tr. R. G. Latham, 2 vols., London, The Sydenham Society, 1848-1850, I, 115.

17. John W. Todd, The errors of medicine, *The Lancet*, 1970, *I*, 665-670.

## Chapter 12

1. Louis Martinet, *Manual of pathology*, tr. Jones Quain, 2nd ed., London, W. Simpkin, 1827. The quotation in the paragraph is part of the subtitle.

2. *Ibid.*, pp. 1-7.

3. *Ibid.*, p. 173.

4. Elisha Bartlett, *An essay on the philosophy of medical science*, Philadelphia, Lea and Blanchard, 1844, p. 59; see also Erwin H. Ackerknecht, Elisha Bartlett and the philosophy of the Paris clinical school, *Bull. Hist. Med.*, 1950, 24, 43-60; Lester S. King, Medical philosophy, 1836-1844, in *Medicine, science and culture: historical essays in honor of Owsei Temkin*, ed. Lloyd G. Stevenson and Robert P. Multauf, Baltimore, The Johns Hopkins University Press, 1968, pp. 143-159.

5. Elisha Bartlett, *An introductory lecture on the objects and nature of medical science*, Lexington, Kentucky, Finnell, 1841, pp. 11, 14.

6. Bartlett, *Philosophy of medical science*, p. 59.

7. John M. Eyler, *Victorian social medicine: the ideas and methods of William Farr*, Baltimore, The Johns Hopkins University Press, 1979, p. 16; M. J. Cullen, *The statistical movement in early Victorian Britain: the foundations of empirical social research*, New York, Barnes and Noble, 1975, p. 6.

8. A commentary of 1838, quoted by Eyler, p. 15.

9. Claude Bernard, *An introduction to the study of experimental medicine*, tr. Henry Copley Green, New York, Dover Publications, 1957.

10. Carl L. Becker, What are historical facts? in *The philosophy of history in our time: an anthology*, ed. Hans Meyerhoff, New York, Doubleday and Co., 1959, pp. 120-137.

11. David Hackett Fischer, *Historians' fallacies: towards a logic of historical thought*, New York, Harper and Row, 1970, p. xv, note.

12. Allan J. Lichtman and Valerie French, *Historians and the living past: the theory and practice of historical study*, Arlington Heights, Illinois, A H M Publishing Corporation, 1978, p. 42; Patrick Gardiner, *The nature of historical explanation*, Oxford, Oxford University Press, 1952, p. 80.

## Chapter 13

1. (Bernard le Bovier de Fontanelle), *The history of oracles and the cheats of the pagan priests*, London, 1688 (facsimile), pp. 21-22, in *The achievement of Bernard le Bovier de Fontanelle*, with introduction by Leonard M. Marsak, New York, Johnson Reprint Corporation, 1970 (original pagination preserved).

2. Lester S. King, *The road to medical enlightenment, 1650-1695*, New York, American Elsevier Inc., 1970.

3. Francis Bacon, *The new organon, or true directions concerning the interpretation of nature*, Book II, aphorism 39, in *The new organon and related writings*, ed. Fulton H. Anderson, New York, The Liberal Arts Press, 1960, p. 206.

4. Bacon, *The great instauration*, in *The new organon*, ed. Anderson. p. 22.

5. *Ibid.*, p. 14.

6. Bacon, *The new organon*, Book I, aphorism 95, Anderson, p. 93.

7. *Ibid.*, Book I, aphorism 46, Anderson, p. 50.

8. *Ibid.*, aphorisms 103-104, Anderson, pp. 97-98.

9. *Ibid.*, aphorism 70, Anderson, p. 67.

10. King, *Road to medical enlightenment*, pp. 62-86.

11. Robert Boyle, *Of the usefulness of natural philosophy*, Part II, in *The works of the honourable Robert Boyle*, 6 vols., London, W. Johnston et al, 1772 (facsimile reprint, Hildesheim, Georg Olms, 1966), II, 195, 97. No one, I believe, has previously pointed out that the five "essays" in this work correspond to the five divisions of the traditional "Institutes of Medicine," namely, physiology, pathology, semeiotics, hygiene, and therapeutics. Except for the reference to page 97, above, the quotations are all from the fifth essay, dealing with therapeutics.

12. Boyle, II, 131.

13. *Ibid.*, pp. 145-146.

14. Lester S. King, *The growth of medical thought*, Chicago, University of Chicago Press, 1963, p. 46.

15. *Galen, on the usefulness of the parts of the body*, tr. Margaret Tallmadge May, 2 vols., Ithaca, New York, Cornell University Press, I, 119.

16. John Farquhar Fulton, *Vesalius four centuries later*, Lawrence, Kansas, University of Kansas Press, 1950, pp. 17-18.

17. *Ibid.*, p. 22.

18. Alan Gregg, Humanism and science, *Bull. N.Y. Acad. Med.*, 1941, *17*, 63-99.

19. Thomas Percival, *Essays medical and experimental*, 2nd ed., London, J. Johnson, 1772 (first ed., 1758), pp. 3-37.

20. *Ibid.*, pp. 41-54.

21. Francisco Boissier de Sauvages, *Nosologia methodica sistens morborum classes juxta Sydenhami mentem et botanicorum ordinem*, 2nd ed., 2 vols., Amsterdam, de Tournes, I, 8 (Prolegomena, par. 19), my translation.

22. Lester S. King, *The medical world of the eighteenth century*, Chicago, University of Chicago Press, 1958, p. 43, pp. 39-44.

23. George Cheyne, *The natural method of cureing the diseases of the body and the disorders of the mind depending on the body*, London, Strahan et al., 1742, pp. 223-224 (capitalization and spelling modernized and italics omitted); Lester S. King, George Cheyne, mirror of eighteenth century medicine, *Bull. Hist. Med.*, 1974, *48*, 517-539.

24. James Lind, *A treatise of the scurvy* (Edinburgh, Sands, Murray and Cochran, 1753), reprinted in *Lind's treatise on scurvy*, ed. C. P. Stewart and Douglas Guthrie, Edinburgh, The University Press, 1953, pp. 145-148.

25. Ulrich Troehler, *Quantification in British medicine and surgery, 1750-1830, with special reference to its introduction into therapeutics*, Dissertation for the degree of doctor of philosophy in the University of London, University College, un-

published. I am greatly indebted to Dr. William Bynum for calling this dissertation to my attention and providing me with a copy.

26. John Stuart Mill, *A system of logic, ratiocinative and inductive*, 2 vols., 2nd ed., London, John W. Parker, 1846, I, 345-533.

27. P. Ch. A. Louis, *Researches on the effects of bloodletting in some inflammatory diseases*, tr. C. G. Putnam, Boston, Hilliard, Gray and Co., 1836.

28. Harry F. Dowling, *Fighting infection: conquests of the twentieth century*, Cambridge, Massachusetts, Harvard University Press, 1977, p. 77.

29. Mill, *System of logic*, I, 455-456.

30. Francis Bacon, *Sylva sylvarum: or a natural history*, in *The works of Francis Bacon*, ed., James Spedding, Robert Leslie Ellis, and Douglas Denon Heath, 14 vols., London, Longman et al., 1857-1874 (facsimile reprint, Stuttgart, Fromann Verlag, 1963) (Century IX), II, 602.

## Chapter 14

1. Abraham Flexner, *Medical education in the United States and Canada: A report to the Carnegie Foundation for the Advancement of Teaching*, Bulletin number four, New York, The Carnegie Foundation for the Advancement of Teaching, 1960 (facsimile of original 1910 edition). The quotations given *infra* are found on pages 52-56.

2. Ludwig W. Eichna, Medical-school education, 1975-1979: A Student's perspective, *New Engl. J. Med.*, 1980, *303*, 727-734.

3. Herman Boerhaave, *Praelectiones academicae*, 5 vols., Turin, Typographia Regia (par. 24 and note *ratiocinatio*), I, 42, my translation. The standard English translation, *Academical lectures on the theory of physic*, 6 vols., London, Rivington et al., 1751-1757, is not sufficiently accurate in these passages.

4. Thomas Reid, *An essay on the nature and cure of the phthisis pulmonalis*, London, T. Cadell, 1782. The quotations are taken from Chapters 4 and 5, pp. 32-44.

5. I am greatly indebted to Professor Kenneth F. Schaffner for permission to study his as yet unpublished manuscript, Problems in computer diagnosis; and for the valuable reference, Edward H. Shortliffe, Bruce G. Buchanan, and Edward A. Feigenbaum, Knowledge engineering for medical decision-making: a review of computer-based clinical decision aids, *Proc. Inst. Electrical and Electronic Engineers*, 1979, *67*, 1207-1224.

6. I Kings 19: 11 and 12.

# INDEX

abstractions, 193, 251
Achilles, 202
acrimony, 27-29, 101, 194, 231
"action" of the vessels, 230-231
Adams, Robert, 135, 157
Addison, Thomas, 135
Albutt, Sir Clifford, v, 137
Alison, W. P., 238-241
analogy, 56, 58, 271, 300
Ancell, Henry, 47
Andral, Gabriel, 41, 42
apothecaries, 306-308
Arber, Agnes, 116
Archeus, 179, 180
Aristotle, 8, 175, 182, 191; and four
    causes, 204-205; and definitions,
    223
Astruc, Jean, 101, 102
Auenbrugger, Leopold, 82
authority, 268, 273, 275, 278-279
automation, *see* computer

Bacon, Francis, 96, 269-271, 283,
    287-288
bacteria, 180
Baglivi, George, 118
Baker, John R., 37
balance, 209, 211-212
Bartlett, Elisha, 249-250
Basedow, K. A. von, 158
Bassi, Agostino, 60
Bauhin, Gaspard, 113
Bayle, G.-L., 31-34, 46, 50, 55,
    167, 217
Becker, Carl, 255, 256
Beeson, P. B. and McDermott,
    Walsh, 126-127
belief, 268
Bellini, Lorenzo, 280

Bennett, J. H., 47; and blood letting,
    238-241
Berkeley, George, 283
Bernard, Claude, v, 252, 317
Bichat, Xavier, 31, 102, 172
blastema, 39-43, 45-52, 217
blood letting, 14, 227-244; and tu-
    berculosis, 23; and Louis, 116; ra-
    tionale in 18th century, 229-233;
    rationale in 19th century, 234-241
Boerhaave, Herman: and signs, 79,
    99; and experience, 80; and diag-
    nosis, 96-97; and disease, 134; and
    explanation, 197-198; and causa-
    tion, 206, 208; and blood letting,
    229-231, 280, 293, 300; critical
    attitude in, 302
Borelli, G. A., 280
Boyle, Robert, 181-182, 272-275
Bretonneau, Pierre, 135
Bright, Richard, 135, 159, 160
Broussais, F.-J.-V., 31
Brown, John, 232-233
Browning, Robert, vi, vii

cancer: and blastema, 42, 45, 47, 51-
    52; and caseation, 54; silent, 170;
    of breast, 100-103, 173-174; as
    predisposing cause, 200; of thyroid,
    313
caseation (*see* scrofula), 50-54
catarrh, 24, 26-28, 33, 78
cause: general discussion, 187-223;
    Villemin, 57; Koch, 63-64; multi-
    ple factors in, 187-188; relevance
    to, 190; intercalated, 197-199; con-
    comitant, 199-200; antecedent,
    200-202; partial, 200; precipitat-
    ing, 200; causal network, 203; of

cause: general discussion (*cont.*)
  disease, 204-223; kinds of, 205-
  206; linguistic problems in, 205-
  206, 222-223; remote, 207-212;
  proximal, 207-212, 219-220; hidden, 280
cell theory, 37-39, 102
cellular tissue, 39-40
Celsus, 197
Cheyne, George, 283-284
classification (*see* nosology), 105-127;
  kinds of, 105-106; artificial, 106-
  107, 113; of plants, 107-119; natural, 113; and enumeration, 114-
  115; bad c., 115; based on symptoms, 119-123, 124; modern c.,
  123-127
clinical entity, 19, 240; nature of,
  147-153; contrast with disease entity, 149-150, 152; infectious disease
  as, 153-156; non-infectious disease
  as, 157-160
clinical science, 295-296
Clutterbuck, Henry, 228, 234-235
Cohn, Ferdinand, 61
computer, 304-308
consumption, *see* tuberculosis
controls, 270, 272, 275, 283-287,
  303
correlation, 29-30, 122, 194-197
Corvisart, J.-N., 82
crisis, 165, 304
critical judgment, 14; lack of, 121;
  and blood letting, 242-243; in examinations, 291; in scientific
  method, 303-304; and computers,
  305, 307-309
Cullen, William: and consumption,
  18, 25-29, 31; and scrofula, 44;
  and specificity, 56; and acrimony,
  29, 217; and blood letting, 230-
  232, 233; and discrimination, 290-
  291
cults, medical, 297

Da Costa, J. M., 87-88, 89, 90
death: cause of, 212-216; certificate,
  213-214; cell d., 214; brain d.,
  215
definition, 209, 210, 223
Deidier, Antoine, 79
Delafield, Francis, and Pruden,
  T. M., 102-103
diagnosis, 90-104; physical, 82; definitions of, 91, 94; framework for,
  92-93; computer d., 96; non-reflective d., 97-98; usefulness of d.,
  103-104
Dioscorides, 108
discrepancy, 278-279, 301-303
discrimination, 102, 155, 301, 304;
  d. between pus and mucus, 289-
  292
disease (*see* health; causes): nature of,
  165-183; causes of, 187-203, 205-
  223; classification of, 173; d. entity, 122, 167; as opposite of health,
  131-132; concept influenced by cultural factors, 137-139, 144-145;
  threatening life vs. impairing comfort, 140-142; role of pain in, 143-
  145
disease entity: "knowledge about,"
  148, 150-152; contrast with clinical
  entity, 149-150; nature of, 151; tuberculosis as a, 153-154; malaria as
  a, 154-155; puerperal fever as a,
  155-156; non-infectious states as,
  157-160
dissection, 277
Dorland's dictionary, 89
Dowling, Harry F., 286

empiricism (empirical), 30, 191,
  247, 275; and Percival, 279-280;
  and Flexner Report, 298; and automation, 308; and "scientific medicine," 309
Enlightenment, 69, 267-268

evaluation, 300-301, 304-305, 307, 317

events: and traces, 253-257, 312-314; reconstruction of, 256-257

evidence: and scientific method, 271, 272, 274, 287, 289; evaluation of, 292-293; acceptance of, 316-317

experience, 80, 268, 274, 280-281

experiment, 135-136, 270

explanation, 219, 258-259


facts, 239, 247-266, 313-314; in history, 252-257; in science, 257-259; and theory, 259-261; "bare" facts, 263-264; establishing facts, 264-265

Fernel, Jean, 77, 79, 300

Fischer, D. H., 255

Fitzgerald, Edward, 253

Flexner, Abraham, 297-298, 303, 306

Flexner Report, 297-299

Fontanelle, B. Le Bovier de, 267-268

form, 182-183

fracture, 207, 209-210

French, Valerie, 259

Fulton, John F., 277-278


Galen (Galenic), 12, 77, 78, 132, 172, 181, 197, 200, 276, 300

Gardner, Patrick, 257

generalization, 258-259, 271, 281-282, 305

genus and species, 106-107

Gesner, Conrad, 111

Gladstone, W. E., 258

Glanders, 57-58

God, 182, 267, 268, 270, 314-315

gout, 170

Graves, Robert, 158-159

Gregg, Alan, 279

Gregory, John (and James), 238

Guttentag, Otto, 152

health: descriptive and normative aspects of, 132-133; relation to function, 133-137; statistics as defining, 139-140

Hegel, G.W.F., 315

Helmont, J. B. van, 179, 273

hemoptysis, 28

Henle, Jacob, 60, 62

herbal, 109, 114

Hippocrates, 22, 80, 151, 195, 196, 282; and clinical entities, 154, 155; and blood letting, 227-228

history: teaching of medical h., 12-13; h. as particularity, 189; as "facts," 252-254; historical events, 255-257; h. and individuals, 255, 258; and traces, 253-257; as reconstructing, 257

Hodgkin, Thomas, 135

Hoffmann, Friedrich, 133

holistic medicine, 315-316

Hooke, Robert, 37

Hunter, John, 41

Huntington's chorea, 175

Huxley, Thomas, 279

hypertension, 124-125

hypothesis, 247, 252, 280-281


idols, 271

immaterial, the, 179

immunology, 21, 65-69

infections, 165, 170, 199; latent, 169

inference, 79-80, 82-85, 100, 178, 193, 281-282, 288, 292

inflammation, 23, 197, 198; and blood letting, 229-232, 235-237, 241

institutes of medicine, 77

interpretation, 82-87, 288-290


jaundice, 125

Jenner, Edward, 293

Jevons, W. S., 94-95

Joyce, James, 255
Julius Caesar, 255, 257-258

Koch, Robert, 48, 54; and tubercle
  bacillus, 60-65, 218; "Koch phenomenon," 65-67; K.'s postulates,
  63
Kramer, Cecile E., vii

Laennec, R.-T.-H., 31, 34-35, 46,
  50, 55, 82, 135, 217
Landré-Beauvais, A.-J., 79
Lebert, Hermann, 52, 56
Leeuwenhoek, Anton van, 269
Lichtman, Allen J. and French, Va-
  lerie, 259
Lind, James, 284-285
Linnaeus, Carolus, 110, 116-117
Lister, Joseph, 60
Louis, P.-C.-A., 31, 135, 166, 285

Malpighi, Marcello, 269
Mandelbaum, Maurice, 222-223
Martinet, Louis, 248-249
matter, 183
meaning (interpretation), 80-83, 86-
  87, 121, 147, 262-263
medical heritage, 9, 11, 12
medical progress, 7, 8
microscopy, 35-39, 44, 48, 102, 269
Mill, John Stuart, 206-207, 285-286
miracle, 267
monocausation, 204-205
Morgagni, G. B., 171
Morton, Richard, 18-25, 26, 29, 31,
  56, 160, 219

necessity, 201, 211, 218-220
neogalenic (neogalenist), 77, 179, 191
Niebyl, Peter, 177
Noguchi, Hideyo, 220-221, 316
nominalism, 177, 180
non-naturals, 198

nosology, 25, 110; 18th century n.,
  117-123; present-day n., 123-127

ontology, 175-183
Osler, William, 293

Pagel, Walter, 177
Paracelsus, 179
paradox, 311
Parkinson, John, 114-115, 127
pattern: in tuberculosis, 16, 57; in diagnosis, 98; in meteorology, 146-
  147; and theory, 152; and disease
  entities, 160-161; reality of, 181,
  183; in scientific method, 282-283,
  293
perception, 287-288
Percival, Thomas, 279-280
persistent problems, 10
phlebotomy, see blood letting
phthisis, see tuberculosis
Pinel, Philippe, 31, 155-156
Pitcairn, Archibald, 280
Plato, 181, 182
pneumonia, 21, 29, 78, 166, 238-
  241
poliomyelitis, 311-312
Portal, Antoine, 31
precision, 269, 275, 289
pus (see scrofula, blastema), 26-27,
  31, 45-46, 48-49, 52, 54

qualities, 22, 105, 176, 181

Rather, Lelland J., 177
rational, rationalism, 30, 247, 270,
  275, 280-281
Ray, John, 116
reality: and ontology, 176-183; and
  "facts," 265-266; and events, 313-
  314; and truth, 318
reason, 80, 280-281, 302, 304
Reid, Thomas, 302-303

relationship, 181, 182, 183, 193, 195

relativism, 317-318

religion, 267

Risse, Guenter B., 241

Riverius, Lazar, 206

Rokitansky, Carl, 48

Royal Society, 271, 273

Rush, Benjamin, 14, 227, 233

Sarton, George, 276

Sauvages, Francisco Boissier de, 117-127, 281

Schleiden, M. J., 38

Schwann, Theodor, 38-39, 42, 45

science: and causes, 191-192; and classes, 258; and theory, 259-261; laws in s., 259-261; Bacon and, 269; essence of, 289; as technology, method, knowledge, 294-295; distinguished from practice, 296-298; and holism, 315-316

scientific medicine, 6, 294-309

scientific method, 243-244, 264-266, 267-293; and general practice, 301

Scirrhus, 100-102

scrofula, 24-25, 27, 36, 43-44; Ancell, 47-48; Villemin, 59-60; Virchow, 53-54; Koch, 62-64

scurvy, 284-285

Sennert, Daniel, 77, 132-133, 191, 300

signs, 73-89; definition of, 75-76; different kinds of, 80-81, 87; as interpretation, 89, 288; pathognomonic, 99-100

Socrates, 112

soul, 179

specificity, 21, 56, 59, 217-218

spirochetal jaundice, 221

Stahl, G. E., 179, 280

statistics, 139-140, 166, 251-252, 285-286, 300

Stedman's *Dictionary*, 75

Stokes, William, 135, 157

substance, 178

substantial form, 172, 179, 180, 183

van Swieten, G.L.B., 101

Sydenham, Thomas: and classification, 110-112, 113, 116, 117-118; and gout, 152; and blood letting, 243

symptoms, 73-89, 168-170; definition of, 75-76; kinds of, 78; transformation into signs, 81, 100, 123; manifestations of disease, 87-88; evidence, 89; basis for classification, 119-123; and meaning, 122; s. versus disease, 161-162

syndrome, 162-163

syphilis, 57-58

tar water, 283

technician and scientist, 305-306

technology, 69, 288-290, 294-295, 305, 307

Temkin, Owsei, 177

Theophrastus, 108

theory, 192, 193-194, 274-275, 280-281

therapeutics, 242-243, 280, 286

Thomas, Lewis, 10-11

Todd, John W., 244

Tournefort, Joseph, 116

traces (historical): of events, 253-257, 312-313; and patterns, 282

Troehler, Ulrich, 285

tubercle, 20-22, 27-29, 30-31, 33-36; and blastema, 42, 45-48; and causation, 50-54

tuberculosis (*see* tubercle, blastema, pus, scrofula), 15-69, 248-249, 258-259; cause of, 216-220; definitions of, 219-220; gold therapy in, 286; discrimination, 289-290; and Reid, 302-303

typhoid fever, 174

universals, 182, 191

venesection, *see* blood letting
verification, 281
Vesalius, Andreas, 13, 276-278
Villemin, J.-A., 44, 48, 54-60, 218, 258
Virchow, Rudolph: and tuberculosis, 46, 48-54, 55, 102, 180, 217-218; and specificity, 55; and typhus, 213
vitalism, 179

Wardrop, James, 235-237
Washington, George, 227, 228

yellow fever, 220-222

Zimmermann, J. G., 93

*Library of Congress Cataloging in Publication Data*

King, Lester Snow, 1908-
   Medical thinking.  .

   Includes bibliographical references and index.
   1.  Medicine—History.      2.  Medicine—Philosophy.
3.  Tuberculosis—History.    1.  Title.
R131.K48        610'.9      81-11965
ISBN 0-691-08297-9          AACR2

                                        Rev.